Heaven
touches
Earth

Companion

Healing and Deliverance Scriptures and Prayers

Expanded Edition

I0141007

ABOUT THE AUTHOR

Reverend Dr. Derry James-Tannariello is a retired Board Certified Chaplain with the Association of Professional Chaplains. She carries a Doctor of Ministry specializing in Christian Counseling, a Masters of Divinity, an MA in Christian Psychology, a BA in Religion and a BS in Personal Ministries.

Derry founded Chaplain Services at Sierra Nevada Memorial Hospital in California. Hospitals, churches, educational institutions and other community organizations solicit her expertise in training others to minister to the sick and terminally ill, and for help dealing with loss and grief.

Derry is an author and sought-after speaker known for her compassionate heart, humor and life-changing inspirational stories of faith and wisdom. She is an internationally recognized seminar and workshop presenter and an interdenominational guest speaker and lecturer on topics such as "How to Have an Effective Prayer Life," "Personal Transformation," "Relational God," "Spirituality and Health" and many more spiritually uplifting topics.

Derry also speaks and presents seminars on "Spiritual Support in Palliative Care," "Bereavement and Grief," "End of Life," "Ministering to Our Dying Loved Ones," "Effective Hospital Visitation" and other topics in hospital ministry.

Derry resides with her husband part time in New Hampshire and part time in Florida, where she assumes pastoral responsibilities, offers spiritual guidance, chaplain support, and enjoys teaching classes based upon her training and experience.

Derry has authored a number of other books, shown and described at the end of this book. To learn more about her, her other books, or to have her as a speaker for your event, workshop or organization, visit her website:

FreedomInSurrender.net

Or contact her at:

Derry@FreedomInSurrender.net

Heaven touches Earth

Companion

Healing and Deliverance Scriptures and Prayers

Expanded Edition

... I was sick and you visited me; ...
—
Matthew 25:36

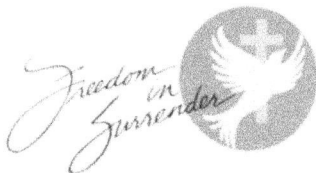

Freedom in Surrender Publishing
Amherst, New Hampshire

Derry James-Tannariello, DMin BCC

Publisher's Cataloging-in-Publication Data
James-Tannariello, Derry
    heaven touches earth companion : healing and
    deliverance scriptures and prayers / by Derry
    James-Tannariello, DMin BCC.—expanded edition
       p. cm.
    ISBN: 978-1-7354208-5-1
    1. Patients-Care. 2. Care-Biblical Teaching.
    3. Chaplains. 4. Caregivers 5. Hospitals-Visitation.
    I. James-Tannariello, Derry. II. Title.

Library of Congress Control Number: 2022909354

ISBN for first edition: 978-1-5146338-4-7

Some of the anecdotal illustrations in this book are true to life and are included with the permission of the persons involved. All other illustrations are composites of real situations, and any resemblance to people living or dead is coincidental.

Printed in the United States of America

Father,

For every patient, we pray that You, Lord, will give them the faith, courage, hope and trust to hold on to You as they go through this challenging journey. We pray peace into their heart, wisdom in their decisions, and gratitude and respect for their caregivers.

In Jesus' name we pray, Amen.

Caring is not a matter of convenience. It is a commitment of one soul to another.
—Susan Staszewski
Keep Your Commitment Strong

And the King will answer and say to them, 'Assuredly, I say to you, inasmuch as you did it to one of the least of these My brethren, you did it to Me.'
—Matthew 25:40

We each, whoever we are, whatever our position, contribute to an environment of care. A love-filled, compassionate and happy individual creates an environment that offers trust, security, hope and healing.
—Derry

DEDICATION

We can only give what is within us. If we, ourselves, are depleted and run down physically, emotionally and/or spiritually, we have little to offer and those we serve suffer from our lack. An empty vessel has nothing to pour out and is more vulnerable to being knocked over and shattered.

This concise reference guide is dedicated to all who long to make a difference in the lives of those suffering, and to all who desire to be effective in hospital, hospice or home ministry—sharing their caring; sharing their love.

Heaven Touches Earth

Father,

For every caretaker, medical practitioner, spiritual representative and business executive, we pray that they will be God-fearing and recognize that they are accountable to You for each decision and act according to Proverbs 9:10.

May they be granted wisdom, knowledge and understanding according to Your promise in James 1:5.

May they recognize their own inadequacies and pray and seek the will of God. (Proverbs 3:58, Luke 11:9)

May they have thankful and teachable spirits (Romans 1:21), and seek pastoral care and counsel when needed. (Hebrews 13:7)

May they be given godly counsel and God-fearing advisors. (Proverbs 24:6)

May they have the courage to resist manipulation, pressure, and the fear of man. (Proverbs 29:25, 2 Timothy 1:7)

May they be generous and have compassionate hearts for the poor and needy. (Psalm 112:9, Luke 10:33-37)

May they be timely, reliable, and dependable. (Matthew 21:28-31)

May they be honest and faithful to their spouses and children. (Malachi 2:15-16)

Help them to be prepared to give account to Almighty God. (Hebrews 9:27)

We pray all of this in the precious and holy name of Jesus the Lord, Amen.

(Taken from *30 Ways to Pray For People In Authority* by Gary P. Bergel)

Contents

Contents

Contents

Contents

Heaven Touches Earth Companion

Contents

Heaven Touches Earth Companion

PREFACE

When we visit a sick, suffering or troubled friend or family member and are at a loss as to what to say, we can turn to God. He knows the heart and needs of each of us and will give us exactly the right words to be effective. One way we can be equipped is to know ahead which scripture promises are applicable to the condition of the one we are visiting.

This book is taken from my more extensive book *Heaven Touches Earth, Expanded Edition.* It is a smaller, easier-to-pack edition of the compilation of scripture and ministry ideas to use in encouraging and bringing relief to those who are suffering. With its extended diversified scriptural resource, care and service suggestions, we pray that all readers will find it more useful.

For more specific instructions as to how to minister and support those of various populations in particular situations or conditions please refer to my book *Heaven Touches Earth, Handbook for Supporting Sick, Terminally Ill and Dying, Expanded Edition.* The topics covered include ministering to patients who are: Young Adults, Adults, Children, Parents, Elderly, Disabled, Blind, and those in Intensive Care/Emergency Room, Surgical Waiting, the Comatose, Chronically Ill, Serious Illness, Critically or Terminally Ill or to the Dying and Bereaved. You will also find a chart listing physical changes and changes in behavior when dying.

It is our hope that both these books will become valuable resources to you and to your friends or colleagues.

And just as you want men to do to you, you also do to them likewise.—Luke 6:31

There are many ways to reach a person's soul. It is in trusting God to reveal the most effective way for each who we encounter, that makes us successful and the patient hopeful and accepting of their future, wherever that may lead.
　　　　　　　　　　—Derry

If any of you lacks wisdom, let him ask of God, who gives to all liberally and without reproach, and it will be given to him.—James 1:5

ACKNOWLEDGMENT

My deepest gratitude to Ray Fusci, my friend and editor who has worked tirelessly to help me compile and prepare this expanded *Companion* edition. May God continue to use his talents for Kingdom glory, and refresh and bless him in all his endeavors. He is my gift from God.

A stranger is a friend we have not met yet. When we have, if we can let them into our heart, they may become our best friend and greatest treasure. Look at every person as priceless, and let God reveal to you their heart.

—Derry

There is power in declaring God's Word.
Jesus Himself used scripture to confront the
challenges He faced. If that was His weapon,
so it should be ours—as well as our hope,
confidence and peace.
—Derry

*So then faith comes by hearing, and hearing by the
Word of God.*—Romans 10:17

Jesus came to deliver men from sin and sickness that He might make known the love of
the Father. In His actions, in His teaching of
the disciples, and the work of the apostles,
pardon and healing are always found together.
—Andrew Murray,
Divine Healing

HEALING AND DELIVERANCE SCRIPTURES AND PRAYERS

> Prayer is our primary lifeline to God. If
> God's life is to flow into us and through us
> into the world, we must be people of prayer.
> —Roy Lawrence,
> *The Practice of Christian Healing*

Prayer/Claiming Bible Promises

Prayer should be offered after you have had a
meaningful interaction with the person, and
have explored areas of concern and importance.
In a crisis situation, prayer, readings, or claiming
scripture promises, can be calming, emphasizing
the resources of peace, strength, courage, quietness, fellowship and hope. It is also healing to
hold hands when praying. With many Christian
groups, comfort is found in repeating the Lord's
Prayer together. Form a prayer circle around the
bed with family, holding hands to bring unity to
the attendees. (For your own protection and
health, be sure to wash your hands after ministering.)

Misuse:

Prayer can be used in a way of providing the
simple solution to a complex problem, shifting
all responsibility to God instead of allowing the
patient to investigate their need to make lifestyle
adjustments. Unfortunately, some are tempted
to use prayer to preach something they feel un-

able to address directly. This is inappropriate. Prayer is also used to help make a graceful exit because there is a sense that it is expected. Don't feel you have to pray. Follow the lead of the Holy Spirit.

Positive applications:

Prayer should present to God the feelings and perspectives of the patient, without judgment. It should make a place for negative feelings. Prayer can release buried emotions so healing can take place. Prayer, shared with discernment, can assist in giving reinforcement for the "will to live" and help break the cycle of pain, bringing comfort and strength.

Applying scripture as we pray, incorporating the healing, protective, caring promises of God, is one of the greatest gifts towards peace. Submitting the patient's future for God to fulfill His destiny in their life, can bring them calm and peace not of this world.

Suggested application:

To work together with God for healing or comfort, one should begin their prayers with praise. In offering the Prayer of Faith, we see that scripture teaches that praise dispels the enemy and gives us access to heaven. God inhabits the praises of His people. Next we are to offer confessions and ask for forgiveness (James 5:16, 1 John 1:9). Now present your intercession, your supplications/requests before God (Matthew 7:7-8), thanking Him in advance for His answers (Philippians 4:6). As you pray, mention scriptural promises, reminding God of what He has done in the past. Prayer just before leaving can have a positive affect because it will be the last thing said and will be foremost on the patient's mind.

Scripture/Encouraging Readings

Scripture can hinder or help.

Hindrance

The timing, when ministering with scripture, can be critical to the healing and hope for the patient's eternal future. This is not a time for condemnation, but for encouragement and salvation. Using scripture before the patient has had an opportunity to explore the depth of their concerns may be premature. This is especially so if they are intensely and totally absorbed in personal conflicts such as: pain, fear, resentment, hostility, grief, anger, or situational stress. When the time comes to use scripture, if a patient is struggling with their feelings toward God, or is angry with Him, then a more generic reading might be more effective to begin with.

Help

When using scripture as a point of identification, for a source of courage and strength or for comfort, it can help the patient be conscious of God's awareness of their situation. It can also be a diagnostic tool to help you become aware of the deeper heart issues that need addressing. You can instruct, inform, teach, and comfort. Depending on the emotional and spiritual health and current perspective of the patient, it might be more advisable to read an encouraging thought that will give them the comfort, hope, courage and reminder that God is with them. Biblical promises can be incorporated when they are more open to hearing them.

Strength, courage and wisdom for each day is at our fingertips; if we are willing to invest a bit of time and attention in our relationship with God and start our mornings with Him. His word in Matthew 6:33 tells us *But seek first the kingdom of God and His righteousness, and all these things shall be added to you.* It's a matter of getting our priorities in order.

The *Bible* is an inspiring, encouraging, and reassuring resource when dealing with sickness and suffering. There is power in the Word of God. Albeit we don't understand, God has a purpose if He allows sickness and suffering. He cares for our needs and carries our burdens. Pain and suffering can lead us closer to God if we are willing to turn to Him. He answers our "Prayer of Faith" according to His divine will for our eternal destiny. He will give sufficient grace for every trial. Put your trust in the ultimate Source of Life. Apply His promises from Scripture applicable to your needs.

The Scriptures listed here are intended to give you the tools for achievement.

ABANDONMENT

"Can a woman forget her nursing child, And not have compassion on the son of her womb? Surely they may forget, Yet I will not forget you. See, I have inscribed you on the palms of My hands; *your walls* are *continually before Me.*—Isaiah 49:15-16

ABUSE

The LORD has taken away the judgments against you, he has cast out your enemies. The King of Israel, the LORD, is in your midst; you shall fear evil no more. "Behold, at that time I will deal with all your oppressors. And I will save the lame and gather the outcast, and I will change their shame into praise and renown in all the earth. At that time I will bring you home, at the time when I gather you together; yea, I will make you renowned and praised among all the peoples of the earth, when I restore your fortunes before your eyes," says the LORD.
—Zephaniah 3:15, 19-20 RSV

ADDICTIONS/ALCOHOL/DRUGS

And Asa cried out to the LORD his God, and said, "LORD, it is nothing for You to help, whether with many or with those who have no power; help us, O LORD our God, for we rest on You, and in Your name we go against this multitude. O LORD, You are our God; do not let man prevail against You!
—2 Chronicles 14:11

Wine is a mocker, strong drink is a brawler, and whoever is led astray by it is not wise.
—Proverbs 20:1

Who has woe? Who has sorrow? Who has strife? Who has complaining? Who has wounds without cause? Who has redness of eyes? Those who tarry long over wine, those who go to try mixed wine. Do not look at wine when it is red, when it sparkles in the cup and goes down smoothly. At the last it bites like a serpent, and stings like an adder. Your eyes will see strange things, and your mind utter perverse things. You will be like one who lies down in the midst of the sea, like one who lies on the top of a mast. "They struck me," you will say, "but I was not hurt; they beat me, but I did not feel it. When shall I awake? I will seek another drink."
—Proverbs 23:29-35 RSV

They shall not drink wine with a song; Strong drink is bitter to those who drink it.—Isaiah 24:9

ADOPTION

For you did not receive the spirit of bondage again to fear, but you received the Spirit of adoption by whom we cry out, "Abba, Father."—Romans 8:15

AFFLICTIONS

And Jehovah said, I have surely seen the affliction of my people … and have heard their cry … for I know their sorrows; and I am come down to deliver them …—Exodus 3:7-8 ASV

I know that the LORD will maintain The cause of the afflicted, And *justice for the poor. Surely the righteous shall give thanks to Your name; The upright shall dwell in Your presence.*
—Psalm 140:12-13

Surely He has borne our griefs And carried our sorrows; yet we esteemed Him stricken, Smitten by God, and afflicted. But He was *wounded for our transgressions,* He was *bruised for our iniquities; the chastisement for our peace* was *upon Him, And by His stripes we are healed.*—Isaiah 53:4-5

What do you conspire against the LORD? He will make an utter end of it. Affliction will not rise up a second time.—Nahum 1:9

Then His fame went throughout all Syria; and they brought to Him all sick people who were afflicted with various diseases and torments, and those who were demon-possessed, epileptics, and paralytics; and He healed them.—Matthew 4:24

For He healed many, so that as many as had afflictions pressed about Him to touch Him.
—Mark 3:10

And he said to her, "Daughter, your faith has made you well; go in peace, and be healed of your disease."
—Mark 5:34 RSV

and rescued him out of all his afflictions …
—Acts 7:10 RSV

And Peter said to him, "Aeneas, Jesus the Christ heals you. Arise and make your bed." Then he arose immediately.—Acts 9:34

ANKLES

And he took him by the right hand and lifted him up, and immediately his feet and ankle bones received strength. So he, leaping up, stood and walked and entered the temple with them—walking, leaping, and praising God.—Acts 3:7-8

ANXIETY

In the multitude of my anxieties within me, Your comforts delight my soul.—Psalm 94:19

Anxiety in the heart of man causes depression, But a good word makes it glad.—Proverbs 12:25

Say to those who are fearful-hearted, "Be strong, do not fear! Behold, your God will come with vengeance, With the recompense of God; He will come and save you."—Isaiah 35:4

Which of you by worrying can add one cubit to his stature?—Matthew 6:27

But I want you to be without care. He who is unmarried cares for the things of the Lord—how he may please the Lord.—1 Corinthians 7:32

casting all your cares [all your anxieties, all your worries, and all your concerns, once and for all] on Him, for He cares about you [with deepest affection, and watches over you very carefully].
—1 Peter 5:7 AMP

Be anxious for nothing, but in everything by prayer and supplication, with thanksgiving, let your requests be made known to God;—Philippians 4:6

ARTHRITIS

A merry heart does good, like medicine, But a broken spirit dries the bones.—Proverbs 17:22

ASK

'Call to Me, and I will answer you, and show you great and mighty things, which you do not know.'
—Jeremiah 33:3

Likewise the Spirit also helps in our weaknesses. For we do not know what we should pray for as we ought, but the Spirit Himself makes intercession for us with groanings which cannot be uttered.
—Romans 8:26

If any of you lacks wisdom, let him ask of God, who gives to all liberally and without reproach, and it will be given to him.—James 1:5

BACKSLIDING

"I will heal their backsliding, I will love them freely, for My anger has turned away from him.
                    —Hosea 14:4

BARRENNESS/CONCEPTION

But Abram said, "LORD GOD, what will You give me, seeing I go childless …" Then Abram said, "Look, You have given me no offspring; indeed one born in my house is my heir!" And behold, the word of the LORD came to him, saying, "This one shall not be your heir, but one who will come from your own body shall be your heir."—Genesis 15:2-4

So Abraham prayed to God, and God healed Abimelech, his wife, and his female servants. Then they bore children;—Genesis 20:17

"So you shall serve the LORD your God, and He will bless your bread and your water. And I will take sickness away from the midst of you. No one shall suffer miscarriage or be barren in your land; I will fulfill the number of your days.
                    —Exodus 23:25-26

So Boaz took Ruth and she became his wife; and when he went in to her, the LORD gave her conception, and she bore a son.—Ruth 4:13

Then he said, "Hear now, O house of David! Is it a small thing for you to weary men, but will you weary my God also? "Therefore the Lord Himself will give you a sign: Behold, the virgin shall conceive and bear a Son, and shall call His name Immanuel.
                    —Isaiah 7:13-14

They shall not labor in vain, Nor bring forth children for trouble; For they shall be the descendants of the blessed of the LORD, And their offspring with them. "It shall come to pass That before they call, I will answer; And while they are still speaking, I will hear.—Isaiah 65:23-24

BELIEVE

But as many as received Him, to them He gave the right to become children of God, to those who believe in His name:—John 1:12

For God so loved the world that He gave His only begotten Son, that whoever believes in Him should not perish but have everlasting life.—John 3:16

"He who believes in Him is not condemned; but he who does not believe is condemned already, because he has not believed in the name of the only begotten Son of God.—John 3:18

Jesus said to her, "I am the resurrection and the life. He who believes in Me, though he may die, he shall live. And whoever lives and believes in Me shall never die. Do you believe this?"—John 11:25-26

Jesus said to him, "Thomas, because you have seen Me, you have believed. Blessed are *those who have not seen and* yet *have believed.*—John 20:29

To Him all the prophets witness that, through His name, whoever believes in Him will receive remission of sins.—Acts 10:43

So they said, "Believe on the Lord Jesus Christ, and you will be saved, you and your household."
—Acts 16:31

that if you confess with your mouth the Lord Jesus and believe in your heart that God has raised Him from the dead, you will be saved. For with the heart one believes unto righteousness, and with the mouth confession is made unto salvation.
—Romans 10:9-10

But without faith it is impossible to please Him, for he who comes to God must believe that He is, and that He is a rewarder of those who diligently seek Him.—Hebrews 11:6

BLESSED

Blessed are the pure in heart, For they shall see God.—Matthew 5:8

BLIND

In that day the deaf shall hear the words of a book, and out of their gloom and darkness the eyes of the blind shall see.—Isaiah 29:18 RSV

I will bring the blind by a way they did not know; I will lead them in paths they have not known. I will make darkness light before them, And crooked places straight. These things I will do for them, And not forsake them.—Isaiah 42:16

Then one was brought to Him who was demon- possessed, blind and mute; and He healed him, so that the blind and mute man both spoke and saw.
—Matthew 12:22

But blessed are your eyes for they see, and your ears for they hear.—Matthew 13:16

Then great multitudes came to Him, having with them the lame, blind, mute, maimed, and many others; and they laid them down at Jesus' feet, and He healed them.—Matthew 15:30

So Jesus had compassion and touched their eyes. And immediately their eyes received sight, and they followed Him.—Matthew 20:34

Then the blind and the lame came to Him in the temple, and He healed them.—Matthew 21:14

Then He came to Bethsaida, and they brought a blind man to Him, and begged Him to touch him. So He took the blind man by the hand and led him out of the town. And when He had spit on his eyes and put His hands on him; He asked him if he saw anything. And he looked up and said, "I see men like trees, walking." Then He put His hands on his eyes again and made him look up. And he was restored and saw everyone clearly.—Mark 8:22-25

"The Spirit of the LORD is upon Me, Because He has anointed Me To preach the gospel to the poor; He has sent Me to heal the brokenhearted, To proclaim liberty to the captives And recovery of sight to the blind, To set at liberty those who are oppressed.—Luke 4:18

saying to him, "Go, wash in the pool of Silo'am" (which means Sent). So he went and washed and came back seeing.—John 9:7 RSV

BLOOD TRANSFUSION

For the life of the flesh is in the blood, ...
—Leviticus 17:11

BOILS

Now Isaiah had said, "Let them take a lump of figs, and apply it *as a poultice on the boil, and he shall recover."*—Isaiah 38:21

Then Isaiah said, "Take a lump of figs." So they took and laid it *on the boil, and he recovered.*
—2 Kings 20:7

BONES

Have mercy on me, O LORD, for I am *weak; O LORD, heal me, for my bones are troubled.*
—Psalm 6:2

He guards all his bones; Not one of them is broken.
—Psalm 34:20

Make me hear joy and gladness, That *the bones You have broken may rejoice.*—Psalm 51:8

Trust in the LORD with all your heart, And lean not on your own understanding; In all your ways acknowledge Him, And He shall direct your paths. Do not be wise in your own eyes; Fear the LORD and depart from evil. It will be health to your flesh, And strength to your bones.—Proverbs 3:5-8

Pleasant words are like *a honeycomb, sweetness to the soul and health to the bones.*—Proverbs 16:24

A merry heart does good, like *medicine, But a broken spirit dries the bones.*—Proverbs 17:22

Thus says the Lord GOD to these bones: "Surely I will cause breath to enter into you, and you shall live.—Ezekiel 37:5

BREATH

And the LORD God formed man of *the dust of the ground, and breathed into his nostrils the breath of life; and man became a living being.*—Genesis 2:7

The Spirit of God has made me, And the breath of the Almighty gives me life.—Job 33:4

Let everything that has breath praise the LORD. Praise the LORD!—Psalm 150:6

BROKENHEARTED

The LORD *is near to those who have a broken heart, And saves such as have a contrite spirit.*
—Psalm 34:18

He heals the brokenhearted And binds up their wounds.—Psalm 147:3

"The Spirit of the Lord GOD *is upon me, Because the* LORD *has anointed Me To bring good tidings to the poor; He has sent Me to heal the brokenhearted, To proclaim liberty to the captives, And the opening of the prison to* those who are *bound.*
—Isaiah 61:1

BRUISE

Moreover the light of the moon will be as the light of the sun, And the light of the sun will be sevenfold, As the light of seven days, In the day that the LORD *binds up the bruise of His people And heals the stroke of their wound.*—Isaiah 30:26

BURNS

… Take balm for her pain; Perhaps she may be healed.—Jeremiah 51:8

Then I washed you in water; yes, I thoroughly washed off your blood, and I anointed you with oil.—Ezekiel 16:9

CANCER (SEE DISEASES)

COMFORT

The LORD is near to those who have a broken heart, And saves such as have a contrite spirit.
                              —Psalm 34:18

The LORD your God in your midst, The Mighty One, will save; He will rejoice over you with gladness, He will quiet you with His love, He will rejoice over you with singing.—Zephaniah 3:17

Blessed be the God and Father of our Lord Jesus Christ, the Father of mercies and God of all comfort, who comforts us in all our tribulation, that we may be able to comfort those who are in any trouble, with the comfort with which we ourselves are comforted by God.—2 Corinthians 1:3-4

for the Lamb who is in the midst of the throne will shepherd them and lead them to living fountains of waters. And God will wipe away every tear from their eyes.—Revelation 7:17

COMMUNICATING

A soft answer turns away wrath, But a harsh word stirs up anger.—Proverbs 15:1

A wholesome tongue is a tree of life, But perverseness in it breaks the spirit.—Proverbs 15:4

Pleasant words are like a honeycomb, Sweetness to the soul and health to the bones.—Proverbs 16:24

Whoever guards his mouth and tongue Keeps his soul from troubles.—Proverbs 21:23

A word fitly spoken is like apples of gold In settings of silver.—Proverbs 25:11

Words of the wise, spoken quietly, should be heard Rather than the shout of a ruler of fools.
—Ecclesiastes 9:17

but, speaking the truth in love, may grow up in all things into Him who is the head—Christ—
—Ephesians 4:15

For "He who would love life And see good days, Let him refrain his tongue from evil, And his lips from speaking deceit.—1 Peter 3:10

CONTENTMENT

Not that I speak in regard to need, for I have learned in whatever state I am, to be content: I know how to be abased, and I know how to abound. Everywhere and in all things I have learned both to be full and to be hungry, both to abound and to suffer need. I can do all things through Christ who strengthens me.—Philippians 4:11-13

Now godliness with contentment is great gain.
—1 Timothy 6:6

Let your conduct be without covetousness; be content with such things as you have. For He Himself has said, "I will never leave you nor forsake you."
—Hebrews 13:5

CONFIDENCE

For the LORD will be your confidence, And will keep your foot from being caught.—Proverbs 3:26

being confident of this very thing, that He who has begun a good work in you will complete it *until the day of Jesus Christ;*—Philippians 1:6

Let us therefore come boldly to the throne of grace, that we may obtain mercy and find grace to help in time of need.—Hebrews 4:16

So we may boldly say: "The LORD is my helper; I will not fear. What can man do to me?"
—Hebrews 13:6

Now this is the confidence that we have in Him, that if we ask any-thing according to His will, He hears us. And if we know that He hears us, whatever we ask, we know that we have the petitions that we have asked of Him.—1 John 5:14-15

COUNSEL

There are many plans in a man's heart, Nevertheless the LORD's counsel—that will stand.
—Proverbs 19:21

Remember the former things of old, For I am God, and there is no other; I am God, and there is none like Me, Declaring the end from the beginning, And from ancient times things that are not yet done, Saying, 'My counsel shall stand, And I will do all My pleasure,'—Isaiah 46:9-10

COURAGE

Be strong and of good courage, do not fear nor be afraid of them; for the LORD your God, He is the One who goes with you. He will not leave you nor forsake you."—Deuteronomy 31:6

The LORD is my light and my salvation; Whom shall I fear? The LORD is the strength of my life; Of whom shall I be afraid?—Psalm 27:1

Be of good courage, And He shall strengthen your heart, All you who hope in the LORD.
—Psalm 31:24

Whenever I am afraid, I will trust in You. In God (I will praise His word), In God I have put my trust; I will not fear. What can flesh do to me?
—Psalm 56:3-4

Do not be afraid of sudden terror, Nor of trouble from the wicked when it comes; For the LORD will be your confidence, And will keep your foot from being caught.—Proverbs 3:25-26

Fear not, for I am with you; Be not dismayed, for I am your God. I will strengthen you, Yes, I will help you, I will uphold you with My righteous right hand.'—Isaiah 41:10

When you pass through the waters, I will be *with you; And through the rivers, they shall not overflow you. When you walk through the fire, you shall not be burned, Nor shall the flame scorch you. For I* am *the* LORD *your God, The Holy One of Israel, your Savior; …*—Isaiah 43:2-3

Yet in all these things we are more than conquerors through Him who loved us.—Romans 8:37

CRIPPLED

If we are being called to account today for an act of kindness shown to a man who was lame and are being asked how he was healed, But since they could see the man who had been healed standing there with them, there was nothing they could say. For the man who was miraculously healed was over forty years old.—Acts 4:9,14,22 NIV

… a certain man without strength in his feet was sitting, a cripple from his mother's womb, who had never walked. This *man heard Paul speaking. Paul, observing him intently and seeing that he had faith to be healed, said with a loud voice, "Stand up straight on your feet!" And he leaped and walked.*—Acts 14:8-10

CRY

You have heard my voice: "Do not hide Your ear From my sighing, from my cry for help."
—Lamentations 3:56

But You, O LORD, are a shield for me, My glory and the One who lifts up my head. I cried to the LORD with my voice, And He heard me from His holy hill. Selah—Psalm 3:3-4

Blessed be *the LORD, Because He has heard the voice of my supplications!*—Psalm 28:6

Hear my cry, O God; Attend to my prayer. From the end of the earth I will cry to You, When my heart is overwhelmed; Lead me to the rock that is higher than I.—Psalm 61:1-2

O LORD, God of my salvation, I have cried out day and night before You. Let my prayer come before You; Incline Your ear to my cry. For my soul is full of troubles, And my life draws near to the grave.
—Psalm 88:1-3

I cry out with my *whole heart; Hear me, O LORD! I will keep Your statutes. I cry out to You; Save me, and I will keep Your testimonies.*
—Psalm 119:145-146

The LORD *is near to all who call upon Him, To all who call upon Him in truth. He will fulfill the desire of those who fear Him; He also will hear their cry and save them.*—Psalm 145:18-19

"Let not your heart be troubled; you believe in God, believe also in Me.—John 14:1

who, in the days of His flesh, when He had offered up prayers and supplications, with vehement cries and tears to Him who was able to save Him from death, and was heard because of His godly fear,
—Hebrews 5:7

They shall neither hunger anymore nor thirst anymore; the sun shall not strike them, nor any heat; for the Lamb who is in the midst of the throne will shepherd them and lead them to living fountains of waters. And God will wipe away every tear from their eyes."—Revelation 7:16-17

And God will wipe away every tear from their eyes; there shall be no more death, nor sorrow, nor crying. There shall be no more pain, for the former things have passed away."—Revelation 21:4

CURSES TO BLESSINGS

It may be that the LORD *will look on my affliction, and that the* LORD *will repay me with good for his cursing this day."*—2 Samuel 16:12

DEAF

In that day the deaf shall hear the words of a book, and out of their gloom and darkness the eyes of the blind shall see.—Isaiah 29:18 RSV

But blessed are *your eyes for they see, and your ears for they hear;*—Matthew 13:16

And they were astonished beyond measure, saying, "He has done all things well. He makes both the deaf to hear and the mute to speak."—Mark 7:37

DEATH (OF CHILDREN FACING)

Then she went and sat down across from him *at a distance of about a bowshot; for she said to herself, "Let me not see the death of the boy." So she sat opposite* him*, and lifted her voice and wept. And God heard the voice of the lad. Then the angel of God called to Hagar out of heaven, and said to her, "What ails you, Hagar? Fear not, for God has heard the voice of the lad where he* is*. Arise, lift up the lad and hold him with your hand, for I will make him a great nation." Then God opened her eyes, and she saw a well of water. And she went and filled the skin with water, and gave the lad a drink. So God was with the lad; and he grew and dwelt in the wilderness, and became an archer. He dwelt in the Wilderness of Paran; and his mother took a wife for him from the land of Egypt.*

—Genesis 21:16-21

Use with:

But Jesus said, "Let the little children come to Me, and do not forbid them; for of such is the kingdom of heaven."—Matthew 19:14

DEATH (SEE ALSO LIFE)

And he said: "The LORD is my rock and my fortress and my deliverer; The God of my strength, in whom I will trust; My shield and the horn of my salvation, My stronghold and my refuge; My Savior, You save me from violence. I will call upon the LORD, who is worthy to be praised; So shall I be saved from my enemies. "When the waves of death surrounded me, The floods of ungodliness made me afraid. The sorrows of Sheol surrounded me; The snares of death confronted me. In my distress I called upon the LORD, And cried out to my God; He heard my voice from His temple, and my cry entered His ears."—2 Samuel 22:2-7

"Return and tell Hezekiah the leader of My people, Thus says the LORD, the God of David your father: "I have heard your prayer, I have seen your tears; surely I will heal you. On the third day you shall go up to the house of the LORD. And Hezekiah said to Isaiah, "What is the sign that the LORD will heal me, and that I shall go up to the house of the LORD the third day?"
—2 Kings 20:5,8

29

For I know that *my Redeemer lives, And He shall stand at last on the earth; And after my skin is destroyed, this* I know, *That in my flesh I shall see God, Whom I shall see for myself, And my eyes shall behold, and not another.* How *my heart yearns within me!*—Job 19:25-27

O LORD *my God, I cried out to You, and You healed me.*—Psalm 30:2

For this is *God, Our God forever and ever; He will be our guide* Even *to death.*—Psalm 48:14

But God will redeem my soul from the power of the grave, For He shall receive me. Selah
—Psalm 49:15

Blessed be *the Lord,* Who *daily loads us* with benefits, *The God of our salvation!* Selah *Our God* is *the God of salvation; And to* GOD *the Lord* belong *escapes from death.*—Psalm 68:19-20

Who forgives all your iniquities, Who heals all your diseases, Who redeems your life from destruction, Who crowns you with lovingkindness and tender mercies,—Psalm 103:3-4

Their soul abhorred all manner of food, And they drew near to the gates of death. Then they cried out to the LORD in their trouble, And *He saved them out of their distresses. He sent His word and healed them, And delivered* them *from their destructions.*—Psalm 107:18-20

I love the LORD, because He has heard My voice and *my supplications. Because He has inclined His ear to me, Therefore I will call* upon Him *as long as I live. The pains of death surrounded me, And the pangs of Sheol laid hold of me; I found trouble and sorrow. Then I called upon the name of the LORD: "O LORD, I implore You, deliver my soul!" Gracious* is *the LORD, and righteous; Yes, our God* is *merciful. The LORD preserves the simple; I was brought low, and He saved me. Return to your rest, O my soul, for the Lord has dealt bountifully with you. For You have delivered my soul from death, My eyes from tears,* And *my feet from falling. I will walk before the LORD in the land of the living.*—Psalm 116:1-9

I shall not die, but live, And declare the works of the LORD. The LORD has chastened me severely, But He has not given me over to death.
—Psalm 118:17-18

Uphold me according to Your word, that I may live; And do not let me be ashamed of my hope. Hold me up, and I shall be safe, And I shall observe Your statutes continually. Plead my cause and redeem me; Revive me according to Your word.

—Psalm 119:116-117,154

Death and life are *in the power of the tongue, And those who love it will eat its fruit.*

—Proverbs 18:21

He will swallow up death forever, And the Lord GOD will wipe away tears from all faces; The rebuke of His people He will take away from all the earth; For the LORD has spoken. And it will be said in that day: "Behold, this is our God; we have waited for Him, and He will save us. This is the LORD; We have waited for Him; We will be glad and rejoice in His salvation."—Isaiah 25:8-9

The righteous perishes, And no man takes it *to heart; Merciful men* are *taken away, While no one considers That the righteous is taken away from evil. He shall enter into peace; They shall rest in their beds,* Each one *walking* in *his uprightness.*

—Isaiah 57:1-2

"I will ransom them from the power of the grave; I will redeem them from death. O Death, I will be your plagues! O Grave, I will be your destruction! Pity is hidden from My eyes."—Hosea 13:14

And begged Him earnestly, saying, "My little daughter lies at the point of death. Come and lay Your hands on her, that she may be healed, and she will live."—Mark 5:23

So when he heard about Jesus, he sent elders of the Jews to Him, pleading with Him to come and heal his servant. Therefore I did not even think myself worthy to come to You. But say the word, and my servant will be healed. And those who were sent, returning to the house, found the servant well who had been sick.—Luke 7:3,7,10

For God so loved the world that He gave His only begotten Son, that whosoever believes in Him should not perish but have everlasting life.—John 3:16

When he heard that Jesus had come out of Judea into Galilee, he went to Him and implored Him to come down and heal his son, for he was at the point of death.—John 4:47

For I am persuaded that neither death nor life, nor angels nor principalities nor powers, nor things present nor things to come, nor height nor depth, nor any other created thing, shall be able to separate us from the love of God which is in Christ Jesus our Lord.—Romans 8:38-39

who, in the days of His flesh, when He had offered up prayers and supplications, with vehement cries and tears to Him who was able to save Him from death, and was heard because of His godly fear, though He was a Son, yet He learned obedience by the things which He suffered.—Hebrews 5:7-8

Blessed be *the God and Father of our Lord Jesus Christ, who according to His abundant mercy has begotten us again to a living hope through the resurrection of Jesus Christ from the dead,*—1 Peter 1:3

Because you have kept My command to persevere, I also will keep you from the hour of trial which shall come upon the whole world, to test those who dwell on the earth.—Revelation 3:10

Then I heard a voice from heaven saying to me, "Write: 'Blessed are *the dead who die in the Lord from now on.'" "Yes," says the Spirit, "that they may rest from their labors, and their works follow them."*—Revelation 14:13

DEATH, SUPPORTIVE READINGS AT TIME OF

See the section "Ministering Helps."

DECISIONS

Delight yourself also in the LORD, And He shall give you the desires of your heart. Commit your way to the LORD, Trust also in Him, And He shall bring it *to pass.*—Psalm 37:4-5

Trust in the LORD with all your heart, And lean not on your own understanding; In all your ways acknowledge Him, And He shall direct your paths.—Proverbs 3:5-6

A man's heart plans his way, But the LORD directs his steps.—Proverbs 16:9

Thus says the LORD: "Stand in the ways and see, And ask for the old paths, where the good way is, *And walk in it; Then you will find rest for your souls. But they said, 'We will not walk* in it.*
—Jeremiah 6:16

'Call to Me, and I will answer you, and show you great and mighty things, which you do not know.'
—Jeremiah 33:3

Now therefore, thus says the LORD of hosts: "Consider your ways!—Haggai 1:5

If any of you lacks wisdom, let him ask of God, who gives to all liberally and without reproach, and it will be given to him.—James 1:5

DELIVERANCE FROM EVIL

"The Spirit of the Lord GOD is upon Me, because the LORD has anointed Me To preach good tidings to the poor; He has sent Me to heal the broken-hearted, To proclaim liberty to the captives, and the opening of the prison to those who are *bound.*

Isaiah 61:1

Then His fame went throughout all Syria; and they brought to Him all sick people who were afflicted with various diseases and torments, and those who were demon-possessed, epileptics, and paralytics; and He healed them.—Matthew 4:24

When evening had come, they brought to Him many who were demon-possessed. And He cast out the spirits with a word, and healed all who were sick.
—Matthew 8:16

And when He had called His twelve disciples to Him, *He gave them power* over *unclean spirits, to cast them out, and to heal all kinds of sickness and all kinds of disease.*—Matthew 10:1

Heal the sick, cleanse the lepers, raise the dead, cast out demons. Freely you have received, freely give.
—Matthew 10:8

Then one was brought to Him who was demon-possessed, blind and mute; and He healed him, so that the blind and mute man both spoke and saw.
—Matthew 12:22

Then He healed many who were sick with various diseases, and cast out many demons; and He did not allow the demons to speak, be-cause they knew Him.—Mark 1:34

And they cast out many demons, and anointed with oil many who were sick, and healed them.
—Mark 6:13

as well as those who were tormented with unclean spirits. And they were healed.—Luke 6:18

And as he was still coming, the demon threw him down and convulsed him. *Then Jesus rebuked the unclean spirit, healed the child, and gave him back to his father.*—Luke 9:42

Also a multitude gathered from the surrounding cities to Jerusalem, bringing sick people and those who were tormented by unclean spirits, and they were all healed.—Acts 5:16

how God anointed Jesus of Nazareth with the Holy Spirit and with power, who went about doing good and healing all who were oppressed by the devil, for God was with Him.—Acts 10:38

For the weapons of our warfare are not carnal but mighty in God for pulling down strongholds,
—2 Corinthians 10:4

and what is *the exceeding greatness of His power toward us who believe, according to the working of His mighty power which He worked in Christ when He raised Him from the dead and seated* Him *at His right hand in the heavenly* places, *far above all principality and power and might and dominion, and every name that is named, not only in this age but also in that which is to come. And He put all* things *under His feet, and gave Him* to be *head over all* things *to the church, which is His body, the fullness of Him who fills all in all.*
—Ephesians 1:19-23

Having disarmed principalities and powers, He made a public spectacle of them, triumphing over them in it.—Colossians 2:15

DELIVERANCE FROM TROUBLE

Then all this assembly shall know that the LORD does not save with sword and spear; for the battle is the LORD's, and He will give you into our hands. "—1 Samuel 17:47

… Thus says the LORD to you: 'Do not be afraid nor dismayed because of this great multitude, for the battle is *not yours, but God's.*

—2 Chronicles 20:15

Deliverance belongs to the LORD; thy blessing be upon thy people! Selah—Psalm 3:8 RSV

"Because he has set his love upon Me, therefore I will deliver him; I will set him on high, because he has known My name. He shall call upon Me, and I will answer him; I will be *with him in trouble; I will deliver him and honor him.*—Psalm 91:14-15

"For a mere moment I have forsaken you, But with great mercies I will gather you.—Isaiah 54:7

Then Jesus said to those Jews who believed Him, "If you abide in My word, you are My disciples indeed. And you shall know the truth, and the truth shall make you free."—John 8:31-32

Therefore if the Son makes you free, you shall be free indeed.—John 8:36

Now the Lord is the Spirit; and where the Spirit of the Lord is, *there* is *liberty.*—2 Corinthians 3:17

DISABLED

(See also Maimed)

Then great multitudes came to Him, having with them the *lame, blind, mute, maimed, and many others; and they laid them down at Jesus' feet, and He healed them.*—Matthew 15:30

DISCIPLESHIP

Let your light so shine before men, that they may see your good works and glorify your Father in heaven.
—Matthew 5:16

And Jesus came and spoke to them, saying, "All authority has been given to Me in heaven and on earth. Go therefore and make disciples of all the nations, baptizing them in the name of the Father and of the Son and of the Holy Spirit, teaching them to observe all things that I have commanded you; and lo, I am with you always, even to the end of the age." Amen.—Matthew 28:18-20

Then He called His twelve disciples together and gave them power and authority over all demons, and to cure diseases. He sent them to preach the kingdom of God and to heal the sick.—Luke 9:1-2

Now then, we are ambassadors for Christ, as though God were pleading through us: we implore you *on Christ's behalf, be reconciled to God. For He made Him who knew no sin* to be *sin for us, that we might become the righteousness of God in Him.*

—2 Corinthians 5:20-21

DISEASES

and said, "If you diligently heed the voice of the LORD *your God and do what is right in His sight, give ear to His commandments and keep all His statutes, I will put none of the diseases on you which I have brought on the Egyptians; for I am the* LORD *who heals you."*—Exodus 15:26

Therefore you shall keep the commandment, the statutes, and the judgments which I command you today, to observe them. "Then it shall come to pass, because you listen to these judgments, and keep and do them, that the LORD *your God will keep with you the covenant and the mercy which He swore to your fathers. And the* LORD *will take away from you all sickness, and will afflict you with none of the terrible diseases of Egypt which you have known, but will lay them on all those who hate you.*

—Deuteronomy 7:11-12,15

Who forgives all your iniquities, Who heals all your diseases,—Psalm 103:3

And Jesus went about all Galilee, teaching in their synagogues, preaching the gospel of the kingdom, and healing all kinds of sickness and all kinds of disease among the people.—Matthew 4:23

When evening had come, they brought to Him many who were demon-possessed. And He cast out the spirits with a word, and healed all who were sick, that it might be fulfilled which was spoken by Isaiah the prophet, saying: "He Himself took our infirmities And bore our sicknesses."

—Matthew 8:16-17

Then Jesus went about all the cities and villages, teaching in their synagogues, preaching the gospel of the kingdom, and healing every sickness and every disease among the people.—Matthew 9:35

And when He had called His twelve disciples to Him, He gave them power over unclean spirits, to cast them out, and to heal all kinds of sickness and all kinds of disease.—Matthew 10:1

When the sun was setting, all those who had any that were sick with various diseases brought them to Him; and He laid His hands on every one of them and healed them.—Luke 4:40

So when this was done, the rest of those on the island who had diseases also came and were healed.
—Acts 28:9

DISLOCATION

and make straight paths for your feet, so that what is lame may not be dislocated, but rather be healed.
—Hebrews 12:13

DYSENTERY

And it happened that the father of Publius lay sick of a fever and dysentery. Paul went in to him and prayed, and he laid his hands on him and healed him.—Acts 28:8

EMOTIONAL

He heals the brokenhearted And binds up their wounds.—Psalm 147:3

"The Spirit of the Lord GOD is upon Me, Because the LORD has anointed Me To preach good tidings to the poor; He has sent Me to heal the broken-hearted, to proclaim liberty to the captives, and the opening of the prison to those who are bound.
—Isaiah 61:1

"The Spirit of the LORD *is upon Me, Because He has anointed Me To preach the gospel to the poor; He has sent Me to heal the brokenhearted, To proclaim liberty to the captives And recovery of sight to the blind, To set at liberty those who are oppressed;*—Luke 4:18

For I will restore health to you, and your wounds I will heal, says the LORD, *because they have called you an outcast: '… for whom no one cares!'*
—Jeremiah 30:17 RSV

My son, be attentive to my words; incline your ear to my sayings. Let them not escape from your sight; keep them within your heart. For they are life to him who finds them, and healing to all his flesh.
—Proverbs 4:20-22 RSV

There is one whose rash words are like sword thrusts, but the tongue of the wise brings healing.
—Proverbs 12:18 RSV

Behold, I will bring it health and healing; I will heal them and reveal to them the abundance of peace and truth.—Jeremiah 33:6

As for me, I said, "O LORD, *be gracious to me; heal me, for I have sinned against thee!"*
—Psalm 41:4 RSV

and begged Him that they might only touch the hem of His garment. And as many as touched it were made perfectly well.—Matthew 14:36

When the crowds learned it, they followed Him, and He welcomed them and spoke to them of the kingdom of God, and cured those who had need of healing.—Luke 9:11 RSV

Beloved, I wish above all things that thou mayest prosper and be in health, even as thy soul prospereth.—3 John 2 KJV

Hurt that has not been healed:

They have healed the hurt of My people slightly, saying, 'Peace, peace!' when there is no peace. For they have healed the hurt of the daughter of My people slightly, Saying, 'Peace, peace!' When there is no peace.—Jeremiah 6:14,8:11

The New Testament contains a number of scriptures that identify the believer's relationship to God. These are identified as the "In Him" verses. They apply to everyone who has been reconciled to God through faith in Jesus Christ. The truth about you is not what you feel or think or believe; it is what God's word says about you.

All who have received Him as their personal Lord and Savior have been born again by the Spirit and have become a new creation in Christ

Jesus, *Therefore, if anyone* is *in Christ,* he is *a new creation; old things have passed away; behold, all things have become new.*—2 Corinthians 5:17. The reality of this truth must be appropriated by faith if the believer is to live a victorious Christian life. "In Him" verses are not presented here.

ENCOURAGEMENT

LORD, You have heard the desire of the humble; You will prepare their heart; You will cause Your ear to hear,—Psalm 10:17

Cast your burden on the LORD, And He shall sustain you; He shall never permit the righteous to be moved.—Psalm 55:22

For I know the thoughts that I think toward you, says the LORD, thoughts of peace and not of evil, to give you a future and a hope.—Jeremiah 29:11

Therefore comfort each other and edify one another, just as you also are doing.
　　　　　　　　　　—1 Thessalonians 5:11

Now may our Lord Jesus Christ Himself, and our God and Father, who has loved us and given us everlasting consolation and good hope by grace, comfort your hearts and establish you in every good word and work.—2 Thessalonians 2:16-17

ENEMIES

that you may be sons of your Father in heaven; for He makes His sun rise on the evil and on the good, and sends rain on the just and on the unjust. For if you love those who love you, what reward have you? …—Matthew 5:45-46

"But I say to you who hear: Love your enemies, do good to those who hate you, bless those who curse you, and pray for those who spite-fully use you.
—Luke 6:27-28

EPILEPSY

Then His fame went throughout all Syria; and they brought to Him all sick people who were afflicted with various diseases and torments, and those who were demon-possessed, epileptics, and paralytics; and He healed them.—Matthew 4:24

ETERNAL LIFE

For God so loved the world that He gave His only begotten Son, that whoever believes in Him should not perish but have everlasting life.—John 3:16

He who believes in the Son has everlasting life; and he who does not believe the Son shall not see life, but the wrath of God abides on him."—John 3:36

My sheep hear My voice, and I know them, and they follow Me. And I give them eternal life, and they shall never perish; neither shall anyone snatch them out of My hand. My Father, who has given them *to Me, is greater than all; and no one is able to snatch* them *out of My Father's hand.*—John 10:27-29

Jesus said to her, "I am the resurrection and the life. He who believes in Me, though he may die, he shall live. And whoever lives and believes in Me shall never die. Do you believe this?"—John 11:25-26

And this is eternal life, that they may know You, the only true God, and Jesus Christ whom You have sent.—John 17:3

For the wages of sin is *death, but the gift of God* is *eternal life in Christ Jesus our Lord.*
—Romans 6:23

And the world is passing away, and the lust of it; but he who does the will of God abides forever.
—1 John 2:17

And this is the testimony: that God has given us eternal life, and this life is in His Son. He who has the Son has life; he who does not have the Son of God does not have life.—1 John 5:11-12

that having been justified by His grace we should become heirs ac-cording to the hope of eternal life.
—Titus 3:7

EYES (SEE ALSO SIGHT)

But blessed are *your eyes for they see, and your ears for they hear;*—Matthew 13:16

So Jesus had compassion and touched their eyes. And immediately their eyes received sight, and they followed Him.—Matthew 20:34

Then He put His *hands on his eyes again and made him look up. And he was restored and saw everyone clearly.*—Mark 8:25

saying to him, "Go, wash in the pool of Silo'am" (which means Sent). So he went and washed and came back seeing.—John 9:7 RSV

FAITH

For in it the righteousness of God is revealed from faith to faith; as it is written, "The just shall live by faith."—Romans 1:17

So then faith comes *by hearing, and hearing by the word of God.*—Romans 10:17

Fight the good fight of faith, lay hold on eternal life, to which you were also called and have confessed the good confession in the presence of many witnesses.
—1 Timothy 6:12

I have been crucified with Christ; it is no longer I who live, but Christ lives in me; and the life *which I now live in the flesh I live by faith in the Son of God, who loved me and gave Himself for me.*
—Galatians 2:20

Therefore we also, since we are surrounded by so great a cloud of witnesses, let us lay aside every weight, and the sin which so easily ensnares us, *and let us run with endurance the race that is set before us, looking unto Jesus, the author and finisher of* our *faith, who for the joy that was set before Him endured the cross, despising the shame, and has sat down at the right hand of the throne of God.*
—Hebrews 12:1-2

Is anyone among you sick? Let him call for the elders of the church, and let them pray over him, anointing him with oil in the name of the Lord. And the prayer of faith will save the sick, and the Lord will raise him up. And if he has committed sins, he will be for-given.—James 5:14-15

For whatever is born of God overcomes the world. And this is the victory that has overcome the world—our faith.—1 John 5:4

FAITHFUL

For the LORD loves justice, And does not forsake His saints; They are preserved forever, But the descendants of the wicked shall be cut off.
—Psalm 37:28

He stores up sound wisdom for the upright; He is a shield to those who walk uprightly; He guards the paths of justice, And preserves the way of His saints.—Proverbs 2:7-8

Most men will proclaim each his own goodness, But who can find a faithful man? The righteous man *walks in his integrity; His children* are *blessed after him. A king who sits on the throne of judgment Scatters all evil with his eyes. Who can say, "I have made my heart clean, I am pure from my sin"?*
—Proverbs 20:6-9

O LORD, You are my God. I will exalt You, I will praise Your name, For You have done wonderful things; Your counsels of old are faithfulness and truth.—Isaiah 25:1

Through the LORD's mercies we are not consumed, Because His compassions fail not. They are new every morning; Great is Your faithfulness.
—Lamentations 3:22-23

He who calls you is *faithful, who also will do* it.
—1 Thessalonians 5:24

But the Lord is faithful, who will establish you and guard you *from the evil one.*
—2 Thessalonians 3:3

Let us hold fast the confession of our *hope without wavering, for He who promised* is *faithful.*
—Hebrews 10:23

Do not fear any of those things which you are about to suffer. Indeed, the devil is about to throw some *of you into prison, that you may be tested, and you will have tribulation ten days. Be faithful until death, and I will give you the crown of life.*
—Revelation 2:10

FEAR

The LORD is *my light and my salvation; Whom shall I fear? The LORD* is *the strength of my life; Of whom shall I be afraid? When the wicked came against me To eat up my flesh, My enemies and foes, They stumbled and fell. Though an army may encamp against me, My heart shall not fear; Though war may rise against me, In this I* will *be confident.*
—Psalm 27:1-3

I sought the LORD, and He heard me, And delivered me from all my fears.—Psalm 34:4

Whenever I am afraid, I will trust in You. In God (I will praise His word), In God I have put my trust; I will not fear. What can flesh do to me?
—Psalm 56:3-4

Say to those who are fearful-hearted, "Be strong, do not fear! Behold, your God will come with vengeance, With the recompense of God; He will come and save you."—Isaiah 35:4

But immediately Jesus spoke to them, saying, "Be of good cheer! It is I; do not be afraid."
—Matthew 14:27

For you did not receive the spirit of bondage again to fear, but you received the Spirit of adoption by whom we cry out, "Abba, Father."—Romans 8:15

For God has not given us a spirit of fear, but of power and of love and of a sound mind.
—2 Timothy 1:7

FEET

Your garments did not wear out on you, nor did your foot swell these forty years.—Deuteronomy 8:4

Forty years You sustained them in the wilderness; They lacked nothing; Their clothes did not wear out And their feet did not swell.—Nehemiah 9:21

And he took him by the right hand and lifted him *up, and immediately his feet and ankle bones received strength. So he, leaping up, stood and walked and entered the temple with them—walking, leaping, and praising God.*—Acts 3:7-8

FERTILITY

And Abram said, O Lord Jehovah, what wilt Thou give me, seeing I go childless, … And, behold, the word of Jehovah came unto to him, saying, This man shall not be thine heir, but he that will come forth out of thine own bowels shall be thine heir.
—Genesis 15:2,4 ASV

So Abraham prayed to God, and God healed Abimelech, his wife, and his female servants. Then they bore children;—Genesis 20:17

No one shall suffer miscarriage or be barren in your land; I will fulfill the number of your days.
—Exodus 23:26

Therefore you shall keep the commandment, the statutes, and the judgments which I command you today, to observe them. Then it shall come to pass, because you listen to these judgments, and keep and do them, that the LORD your God will keep with you the covenant and the mercy which He swore to your fathers. And He will love you and bless you and multiply you; He will also bless the fruit of your womb and the fruit of your land, … You shall be blessed above all peoples; there shall not be a male or female barren among you or among your livestock.

—Deuteronomy 7:11-14

They shall not labor in vain, Nor bring forth children for trouble; For they shall be the descendants of the blessed of the LORD, And their offspring with them.—Isaiah 65:23

FEVER

But Simon's wife's mother lay sick with a fever, and they told Him about her at once. So He came and took her by the hand and lifted her up, and immediately the fever left her. And she served them.

—Mark 1:30-31

And it happened that the father of Publius lay sick of a fever and dysentery. Paul went in to him and prayed, and he laid his hands on him and healed him.—Acts 28:8

FINANCES

This Book of the Law shall not depart from your mouth, but you shall meditate in it day and night, that you may observe to do according to all that is written in it. For then you will make your way prosperous, and then you will have good success.
—Joshua 1:8

Let them shout for joy and be glad, Who favor my righteous cause; And let them say continually, "Let the LORD be magnified, Who has pleasure in the prosperity of His servant."—Psalm 35:27

He who has a slack hand becomes poor, But the hand of the diligent makes rich.—Proverbs 10:4

The sleep of a laboring man is sweet, Whether he eats little or much; But the abundance of the rich will not permit him to sleep.—Ecclesiastes 5:12

Here is what I have seen: It is *good and fitting* for one *to eat and drink, and to enjoy the good of all his labor in which he toils under the sun all the days of his life which God gives him; for it* is *his heritage.*—Ecclesiastes 5:18

Bring all the tithes into the storehouse, That there may be food in My house, And try Me now in this," *Says the* LORD *of hosts, "If I will not open for you the windows of heaven And pour out for you* such *blessing That* there will *not* be room *enough* to receive it.—Malachi 3:10

He who is *faithful in* what is *least is faithful also in much; and he who is unjust in* what is *least is unjust also in much.*—Luke 16:10

Owe no one anything except to love one another, for he who loves another has fulfilled the law.
—Romans 13:8

For you know the grace of our Lord Jesus Christ, that though He was rich, yet for your sakes He became poor, that you through His poverty might become rich.—2 Corinthians 8:9

And my God shall supply all your need according to His riches in glory by Christ Jesus.
—Philippians 4:19

Let your conduct be without covetousness; be content with such things as you have. For He Himself has said, "I will never leave you nor forsake you."
—Hebrews 13:5

And let our people also learn to maintain good works, to meet urgent needs, that they may not be unfruitful.—Titus 3:14

HELP WITH FINANCES

Borrowing:

Give to him who asks you, and from him who wants to borrow from you do not turn away.
—Matthew 5:42

A good man deals graciously and lends; He will guide his affairs with discretion.—Psalm 112:5

Giving:

The generous soul will be made rich, And he who waters will also be watered himself.
—Proverbs 11:25

The soul of a lazy man desires, and has nothing; But the soul of the diligent shall be made rich.
—Proverbs 13:4

If your enemy is hungry, give him bread to eat; And if he is thirsty, give him water to drink;
—Proverbs 25:21

58

He who gives to the poor will not lack, But he who hides his eyes will have many curses.
—Proverbs 28:27

But when you do a charitable deed, do not let your left hand know what your right hand is doing, that your charitable deed may be in secret; and your Father who sees in secret will Himself reward you openly.—Matthew 6:3-4

Give, and it will be given to you: good measure, pressed down, shaken together, and running over will be put into your bosom. For with the same measure that you use, it will be measured back to you."
—Luke 6:38

So let each one give as he purposes in his heart, not grudgingly or of necessity; for God loves a cheerful giver.—2 Corinthians 9:7

FORGIVENESS

Offenses can leave emotional and spiritual wounds.

please let Your ear be attentive and Your eyes open, that You may hear the prayer of Your servant which I pray before You now, day and night, for the children of Israel Your servants, and confess the sins of the children of Israel which we have sinned against You. Both my father's house and I have sinned. We have acted very corruptly against You, and have not kept the commandments, the statutes, nor the ordinances which You commanded Your servant Moses. Remember, I pray, the word that You commanded Your servant Moses, saying, "If you are unfaithful, I will scatter you among the nations; but if you return to Me, and keep My commandments and do them, though some of you were cast out to the farthest part of the heavens, yet I will gather them from there, and bring them to the place which I have chosen as a dwelling for My name.' Now these are *Your servants and Your people, whom You have redeemed by Your great power, and by Your strong hand.*—Nehemiah 1:6-10

I acknowledged my sin to You, And my iniquity I have not hidden. I said, "I will confess my transgressions to the LORD," *And You forgave the iniquity of my sin.* Selah—Psalm 32:5

Rejoice the soul of Your servant, For to You, O Lord, I lift up my soul. For You, Lord, are *good, and ready to forgive, And abundant in mercy to all those who call upon You.*—Psalm 86:4-5

Who forgives all your iniquities, Who heals all your diseases, Who redeems your life from destruction, Who crowns you with loving kindness and tender mercies,—Psalm 103:3-4

As far as the east is from the west, So far has He removed our transgressions from us.
—Psalm 103:12

"Come now, and let us reason together," Says the LORD, *"Though your sins are like scarlet, They shall be as white as snow; Though they are red like crimson, They shall be as wool.*—Isaiah 1:18

Then behold, they brought to Him a paralytic lying on a bed. When Jesus saw their faith, He said to the paralytic, "Son, be of good cheer; your sins are forgiven you." And at once some of the scribes said within themselves, "This Man blasphemes!" But Jesus, knowing their thoughts, said, "Why do you think evil in your hearts? For which is easier, to say, 'Your sins are forgiven you,' or to say, 'Arise and walk'? But that you may know that the Son of Man has power on earth to forgive sins"—then He said to the paralytic, "Arise, take up your bed, and go to your house." And he arose and departed to his house. Now when the multitudes saw it, they marveled and glorified God, who had given such power to men.—Matthew 9:2-8

"And whenever you stand praying, if you have anything against anyone, forgive him, that your Father in heaven may also forgive you your trespasses. But if you do not forgive, neither will your Father in heaven forgive your trespasses."—Mark 11:25-26

Now then, we are ambassadors for Christ, as though God were pleading through us: we implore you on Christ's behalf, be reconciled to God. For He made Him who knew no sin to be sin for us, that we might become the righteousness of God in Him.
—2 Corinthians 5:20-21

In Him we have redemption through His blood, the forgiveness of sins, according to the riches of His grace—Ephesians 1:7

"This is the covenant that I will make with them after those days, says the LORD: I will put My laws into their hearts, and in their minds I will write them," then He adds, *"Their sins and their lawless deeds I will remember no more."*
—Hebrews 10:16-17

If we say that we have no sin, we deceive ourselves, and the truth is not in us. If we confess our sins, He is faithful and just to forgive us our sins and to cleanse us from all unrighteousness. If we say that we have not sinned, we make Him a liar, and His word is not in us.—1 John 1:8-10

FUTURE

For I know the thoughts that I think toward you, says the LORD, *thoughts of peace and not of evil, to give you a future and a hope.*—Jeremiah 29:11

But as it is written: "Eye has not seen, nor ear heard, Nor have entered into the heart of man The things which God has prepared for those who love Him." But God has revealed them to us through His Spirit. For the Spirit searches all things, yes, the deep things of God.—1 Corinthians 2:9-10

For our citizenship is in heaven, from which we also eagerly wait for the Savior, the Lord Jesus Christ, who will transform our lowly body that it may be conformed to His glorious body, according to the working by which He is able even to subdue all things to Himself.—Philippians 3:20-21

whereas you do not know what will happen tomorrow. For what is your life? It is even a vapor that appears for a little time and then vanishes away. Instead you ought to say, "If the Lord wills, we shall live and do this or that."—James 4:14-15

GENERAL

Now see that I, even I, am He, and there is no God besides Me; I kill and I make alive; I wound and I heal; nor is there any who can deliver from My hand.—Deuteronomy 32:39

So Moses cried out to the LORD, saying, "Please heal her, O God, I pray!"—Numbers 12:13

O LORD my God, I cried out to You, And You healed me.—Psalm 30:2

Who forgives all your iniquities, Who heals all your diseases, Who redeems your life from destruction, Who crowns you with loving kindness and tender mercies,—Psalm 103:3-4

He sent His word and healed them, and delivered them *from their destructions.*—Psalm 107:20

Do not be wise in your own eyes; Fear the LORD and depart from evil. It will be health to your flesh, And strength to your bones.—Proverbs 3:7-8

For they are *life to those who find them, And health to all their flesh.*—Proverbs 4:22

Surely He has borne our griefs And carried our sorrows; Yet we esteemed Him stricken, Smitten by God, and afflicted. But He was *wounded for our transgressions,* He was *bruised for our iniquities; The chastisement for our peace* was *upon Him, And by His stripes we are healed.*—Isaiah 53:4-5

I have seen his ways, and will heal him; I will also lead him, And restore comforts to him And to his mourners. "I create the fruit of the lips: Peace, peace to him who is *far off and to* him who is *near," Says the* LORD, *"And I will heal him."*
—Isaiah 57:18-19

Then your light shall break forth like the morning, Your healing shall spring forth speedily, And your righteousness shall go before you; The glory of the LORD *shall be your rear guard. Then you shall call, and the* LORD *will answer; You shall cry, and He will say, "Here I* am.*' "If you take away the yoke from your midst, The pointing of the finger, and speaking wickedness,*—Isaiah 58:8-9

Heal me, O LORD, *and I shall be healed; Save me, and I shall be saved, For You are my praise.*
—Jeremiah 17:14

For I will restore health to you And heal you of your wounds,' says the LORD, *…*—Jeremiah 30:17

65

Behold, I will bring it health and healing; I will heal them and reveal to them the abundance of peace and truth.—Jeremiah 33:6

But to you who fear My name The Sun of Righteousness shall arise With healing in His wings; And you shall go out And grow fat like stall-fed calves.—Malachi 4:2

And Jesus said to him, "I will come and heal him." The centurion answered and said, "Lord, I am not worthy that You should come under my roof. But only speak a word, and my servant will be healed. Then Jesus said to the centurion, "Go your way; and as you have believed, so *let it be done for you." And his servant was healed that same hour.*
—Matthew 8:7-8,13

When evening had come, they brought to Him many who were demon-possessed. And He cast out the spirits with a word, and healed all who were sick,
—Matthew 8:16

And great multitudes followed Him, and He healed them there.—Matthew 19:2

Now it happened on a certain day, as He was teaching, that there were Pharisees and teachers of the law sitting by, who had come out of every town of Galilee, Judea, and Jerusalem. And the power of the Lord was present *to heal them.*—Luke 5:17

And the whole multitude sought to touch Him, for power went out from Him and healed them *all.*
—Luke 6:19

And He said to her, "Daughter, be of good cheer; your faith has made you well. Go in peace."
—Luke 8:48

So they departed and went through the towns, preaching the gospel and healing everywhere.
—Luke 9:6

But when the multitudes knew it, they followed Him; and He received them and spoke to them about the kingdom of God, and healed those who had need of healing.—Luke 9:11

by stretching out Your hand to heal, and that signs and wonders may be done through the name of Your holy Servant Jesus."—Acts 4:30

Also a multitude gathered from the surrounding cities to Jerusalem, bringing sick people and those who were tormented by unclean spirits, and they were all healed.—Acts 5:16

For the hearts of this people have grown dull. Their *ears are hard of hearing, And their eyes they have closed, Lest they should see with* their *eyes and hear with* their *ears, Lest they should understand with* their *hearts and turn, so that I should heal them."'*—Acts 28:27

67

Now may the God of peace Himself sanctify you completely; and may your whole spirit, soul, and body be preserved blameless at the coming of our Lord Jesus Christ.—1 Thessalonians 5:23

Confess your trespasses to one another, and pray for one another, that you may be healed. The effective, fervent prayer of a righteous man avails much.
—James 5:16

and He Himself bore our sins in His body on the cross, so that we might die to sin and live to righteousness; by His wounds you were healed.
—1 Peter 2:24 NASB

who Himself bore our sins in His own body on the tree, that we, having died to sins, might live for righteousness—by whose stripes you were healed.
—1 Peter 2:24

GOALS

But seek first the kingdom of God and His righteousness, and all these things shall be added to you.—Matthew 6:33

Do you not know that those who run in a race all run, but one receives the prize? Run in such a way that you may obtain it.—1 Corinthians 9:24

Brethren, I do not count myself to have apprehended; but one thing I do, forgetting those things which are behind and reaching forward to those things which are ahead, I press toward the goal for the prize of the upward call of God in Christ Jesus.

—Philippians 3:13-14

that you also aspire to lead a quiet life, to mind your own business, and to work with your own hands, as we commanded you,—1 Thessalonians 4:11

Be diligent to present yourself approved to God, a worker who does not need to be ashamed, rightly dividing the word of truth.—2 Timothy 2:15

GOD—SEEKING HIM

But from there you will seek the LORD your God, and you will find Him if you seek Him with all your heart and with all your soul.

—Deuteronomy 4:29

And those who know Your name will put their trust in You; For You, LORD, have not forsaken those who seek You.—Psalm 9:10

The LORD looks down from heaven upon the children of men, To see if there are any who understand, who seek God.—Psalm 14:2

Seek the LORD while He may be found, Call upon Him while He is near. Let the wicked forsake his way, And the unrighteous man his thoughts; Let him return to the LORD, And He will have mercy on him; And to our God, For He will abundantly pardon.—Isaiah 55:6-7

Then you will call upon Me and go and pray to Me, and I will lis-ten to you. And you will seek Me and find Me, when you search for Me with all your heart. I will be found by you, says the LORD, and I will bring you back from your captivity; I will gather you from all the nations and from all the places where I have driven you, says the LORD, and I will bring you to the place from which I cause you to be carried away captive.—Jeremiah 29:12-14

The LORD is good to those who wait for Him, To the soul who seeks Him.—Lamentations 3:25

"So I say to you, ask, and it will be given to you; seek, and you will find; knock, and it will be opened to you. For everyone who asks receives, and he who seeks finds, and to him who knocks it will be opened.—Luke 11:9-10

But without faith it is impossible to please Him, for he who comes to God must believe that He is, and that He is a rewarder of those who diligently seek Him.—Hebrews 11:6

GOD WILL HEAR

Not a word failed of any good thing which the LORD had spoken to the house of Israel. All came to pass.—Joshua 21:45

if My people who are called by My name will humble themselves, and pray and seek My face, and turn from their wicked ways, then I will hear from heaven, and will forgive their sin and heal their land.—2 Chronicles 7:14

But know that the LORD has set apart for Himself him who is godly; The LORD will hear when I call to Him.—Psalm 4:3

Because He has inclined His ear to me, Therefore I will call upon Him *as long as I live.*
—Psalm 116:2

They shall not labor in vain, Nor bring forth children for trouble; For they shall be *the descendants of the blessed of the LORD, And their offspring with them. "It shall come to pass That before they call, I will answer; And while they are still speaking, I will hear.*—Isaiah 65:23-24

Then you will call upon Me and go and pray to Me, and I will lis-ten to you. And you will seek Me and find Me, *when you search for Me with all your heart. I will be found by you, says the* LORD, …
—Jeremiah 29:12-14

'Call to Me, and I will answer you, and show you great and mighty things, which you do not know.'
—Jeremiah 33:3

Therefore I will look to the LORD; *I will wait for the God of my salvation; My God will hear me.*
—Micah 7:7

"And in that day you will ask Me nothing. Most assuredly, I say to you, whatever you ask the Father in My name He will give you. Until now you have asked nothing in My name. Ask, and you will re-ceive, that your joy may be full.—John 16:23-24

For the eyes of the LORD *are on the righteous, And His ears* are open *to their prayers; But the face of the* LORD *is against those who do evil."*
—1 Peter 3:12

GOD'S FAITHFULNESS

"Therefore know that the LORD *your God, He is God, the faithful God who keeps covenant and mercy for a thousand generations with those who love Him and keep His commandments;*
—Deuteronomy 7:9

Through the LORD*'s mercies we are not consumed, Because His compassions fail not. They are new every morning; Great is Your faithfulness.*
—Lamentations 3:22-23

For the LORD *is good; His mercy is everlasting, And His truth* endures *to all generations.*
—Psalm 100:5

For Your mercy is great above the heavens, And Your truth reaches *to the clouds.*—Psalm 108:4

The works of His hands are *verity and justice; All His precepts* are *sure. They stand fast forever and ever,* And are *done in truth and uprightness.*
—Psalm 111:7-8

For the mountains shall depart And the hills be removed, But My kindness shall not depart from you, Nor shall My covenant of peace be removed," Says the LORD, *who has mercy on you.*
—Isaiah 54:10

God is faithful, by whom you were called into the fellowship of His Son, Jesus Christ our Lord.—1 Corinthians 1:9

But the Lord is faithful, who will establish you and guard you *from the evil one.*

—2 Thessalonians 3:3

If we confess our sins, He is faithful and just to forgive us our sins and to cleanse us from all unrighteousness.—1 John 1:9

GOD'S PRESENCE

And He said, "My Presence will go with you, *and I will give you rest."*—Exodus 33:14

Be strong and of good courage, do not fear nor be afraid of them; for the LORD *your God, He is the One who goes with you. He will not leave you nor forsake you."*—Deuteronomy 31:6

No man shall be able *to stand before you all the days of your life; as I was with Moses, so I will be with you. I will not leave you nor for-sake you.*

—Joshua 1:5

Yea, though I walk through the valley of the shadow of death, I will fear no evil; For You are *with me; Your rod and Your staff, they comfort me.*

—Psalm 23:4

If I take the wings of the morning, And dwell in the uttermost parts of the sea, Even there Your hand shall lead me, And Your right hand shall hold me.—Psalm 139:9-10

The LORD is near to all who call upon Him, To all who call upon Him in truth.—Psalm 145:18

When you pass through the waters, I will be *with you; And through the rivers, they shall not overflow you. When you walk through the fire, you shall not be burned, Nor shall the flame scorch you. For I am the LORD your God, The Holy One of Israel, your Savior; …*—Isaiah 43:2-3

Even to your *old age, I am He, And* even *to gray hairs I will carry* you*! I have made, and I will bear; Even I will carry, and will deliver* you.
—Isaiah 46:4

The LORD has appeared of old to me, saying: "Yes, I have loved you with an everlasting love; Therefore with lovingkindness I have drawn you.
—Jeremiah 31:3

teaching them to observe all things that I have commanded you; and lo, I am with you always, even *to the end of the age." Amen.*
—Matthew 28:20

so that they should seek the Lord, in the hope that they might grope for Him and find Him, though He is not far from each one of us;—Acts 17:27

that by two immutable things, in which it is impossible for God to lie, we might have strong consolation, who have fled for refuge to lay hold of the hope set before us.—Hebrews 6:18

Let your conduct be without covetousness; be content with such things as you have. For He Himself has said, "I will never leave you nor forsake you."
—Hebrews 13:5

GOD'S WILL

Good and upright is the LORD; Therefore He teaches sinners in the way. The humble He guides in justice, And the humble He teaches His way.
—Psalm 25:8-9

In this manner, therefore, pray: Our Father in heaven, Hallowed be Your name. Your kingdom come. Your will be done On earth as it is in heaven.—Matthew 6:9-10

And this is the will of Him who sent Me, that everyone who sees the Son and believes in Him may have everlasting life; and I will raise him up at the last day."—John 6:40

Now we know that God does not hear sinners; but if anyone is a worshiper of God and does His will, He hears him.—John 9:31

And do not be conformed to this world, but be transformed by the renewing of your mind, that you may prove what is *that good and acceptable and perfect will of God.*—Romans 12:2

Grace to you and peace from God the Father and our Lord Jesus Christ, who gave Himself for our sins, that He might deliver us from this present evil age, according to the will of our God and Father, to whom be glory forever and ever. Amen.
—Galatians 1:3-5

In Him also we have obtained an inheritance, being predestined according to the purpose of Him who works all things according to the counsel of His will, that we who first trusted in Christ should be to the praise of His glory.—Ephesians 1:11-12

For this is the will of God, your sanctification: that you should abstain from sexual immorality; that each of you should know how to possess his own vessel in sanctification and honor,
—1 Thessalonians 4:3-4

Rejoice always, pray without ceasing, in everything give thanks; for this is the will of God in Christ Jesus for you. Do not quench the Spirit.
—1 Thessalonians 5:16-19

77

For this is the will of God, that by doing good you may put to silence the ignorance of foolish men—
—1 Peter 2:15

Therefore let those who suffer according to the will of God commit their souls to Him *in doing good, as to a faithful Creator.*—1 Peter 4:19

And the world is passing away, and the lust of it; but he who does the will of God abides forever.
—1 John 2:17

GRACE

And of His fullness we have all received, and grace for grace.—John 1:16

But we believe that through the grace of the Lord Jesus Christ we shall be saved in the same manner as they."—Acts 15:11

But none of these things move me; nor do I count my life dear to my-self, so that I may finish my race with joy, and the ministry which I received from the Lord Jesus, to testify to the gospel of the grace of God.
—Acts 20:24

So now, brethren, I commend you to God and to the word of His grace, which is able to build you up and give you an inheritance among all those who are sanctified.—Acts 20:32

For you know the grace of our Lord Jesus Christ, that though He was rich, yet for your sakes He became poor, that you through His poverty might become rich.—2 Corinthians 8:9

And God is able to make all grace abound toward you, that you, always having all sufficiency in all things, may have an abundance for every good work.—2 Corinthians 9:8

to the praise of the glory of His grace, by which He made us accepted in the Beloved. In Him we have redemption through His blood, the forgiveness of sins, according to the riches of His grace.
—Ephesians 1:6-7

that in the ages to come He might show the exceeding riches of His grace in His *kindness toward us in Christ Jesus. For by grace you have been saved through faith, and that not of yourselves;* it is *the gift of God, not of works, lest anyone should boast.*
—Ephesians 2:7-9

But to each one of us grace was given according to the measure of Christ's gift.—Ephesians 4:7

not by works of righteousness which we have done, but according to His mercy He saved us, through the washing of regeneration and renewing of the Holy Spirit, whom He poured out on us abundantly through Jesus Christ our Savior, that having been justified by His grace we should become heirs according to the hope of eternal life.—Titus 3:5-7

GUIDANCE

You in Your mercy have led forth The people whom You have redeemed; You have guided them *in Your strength To Your holy habitation.*
                          —Exodus 15:13

He makes me to lie down in green pastures; He leads me beside the still waters. He restores my soul; He leads me in the paths of righteousness For His name's sake.—Psalm 23:2-3

Good and upright is *the* LORD; *Therefore He teaches sinners in the way.*—Psalm 25:8

If I take the wings of the morning, And dwell in the uttermost parts of the sea, Even there Your hand shall lead me, And Your right hand shall hold me.—Psalm 139:9-10

The LORD will guide you continually, And satisfy your soul in drought, And strengthen your bones; You shall be like a watered garden, And like a spring of water, whose waters do not fail.
—Isaiah 58:11

HANDS

Then the king answered and said to the man of God, "Please entreat the favor of the LORD your God, and pray for me, that my hand may be restored to me." So the man of God entreated the LORD, and the king's hand was restored to him, and became as before.—1 Kings 13:6

Strengthen the weak hands, and make firm the feeble knees. Say to those who are *fearful-hearted, "Be strong, do not fear! Behold, your God will come* with *vengeance,* With *the recompense of God; He will come and save you."*—Isaiah 35:3-4

Therefore strengthen the hands which hang down, and the feeble knees, and make straight paths for your feet, so that what is lame may not be dislocated, but rather be healed.—Hebrews 12:12-13

HEADACHES

And he said to his father, "My head, my head!" So he said to a servant, "Carry him to his mother." When Elisha came into the house, there was the child, lying dead on his bed. He went in therefore, shut the door behind the two of them, and prayed to the LORD. And he went up and lay on the child, and put his mouth on his mouth, his eyes on his eyes, and his hands on his hands; and he stretched himself out on the child, and the flesh of the child became warm. He returned and walked back and forth in the house, and again went up and stretched himself out on him; then the child sneezed seven times, and the child opened his eyes.—2 Kings 4:19,32-35

HEALING

O LORD my God, I cried out to You, And You healed me.—Psalm 30:2

I said, "LORD, be merciful to me; Heal my soul, for I have sinned against You."—Psalm 41:4

Bless the LORD, O my soul, And forget not all His benefits: Who forgives all your iniquities, Who heals all your diseases,—Psalm 103:2-3

He sent His word and healed them, And delivered them *from their destructions.*—Psalm 107:20

But He was wounded for our transgressions, He was bruised for our iniquities; The chastisement for our peace was upon Him, And by His stripes we are healed.—Isaiah 53:5

I have seen his ways, and will heal him; I will also lead him, And restore comforts to him And to his mourners. "I create the fruit of the lips: Peace, peace to him who is *far off and to* him who is *near," Says the LORD, "And I will heal him."*
—Isaiah 57:18-19

Heal me, O LORD, and I shall be healed; Save me, and I shall be saved, For You are my praise.
—Jeremiah 17:14

For I will restore health to you And heal you of your wounds,' says the LORD, 'Because they called you an outcast saying: "This is Zion; No one seeks her."'—Jeremiah 30:17

Behold, I will bring it health and healing; I will heal them and reveal to them the abundance of peace and truth.—Jeremiah 33:6

'I will heal their backsliding, I will love them freely, For My anger has turned away from him.
—Hosea 14:4

The centurion answered and said, "Lord, I am not worthy that You should come under my roof. But only speak a word, and my servant will be healed. Then Jesus said to the centurion, "Go your way; and as you have believed, so let it be done for you." And his servant was healed that same hour.

—Matthew 8:8,13

Then great multitudes came to Him, having with them the *lame, blind, mute, maimed, and many others; and they laid them down at Jesus' feet, and He healed them.*—Matthew 15:30

And these signs will follow those who believe: In My name they will cast out demons; they will speak with new tongues; they will take up serpents; and if they drink anything deadly, it will by no means hurt them; they will lay hands on the sick, and they will recover."—Mark 16:17-18

And the prayer of faith will save the sick, and the Lord will raise him up. And if he has committed sins, he will be forgiven. Confess your trespasses to one another, and pray for one another, that you may be healed. The effective, fervent prayer of a righteous man avails much.—James 5:15-16

who Himself bore our sins in His own body on the tree, that we, having died to sins, might live for righteousness—by whose stripes you were healed.

—1 Peter 2:24

HEALTH

Do not be wise in your own eyes; Fear the LORD and depart from evil. It will be health to your flesh, and strength to your bones.—Proverbs 3:7-8

My son, give attention to my words; Incline your ear to my sayings. Do not let them depart from your eyes; Keep them in the midst of your heart; For they are life to those who find them, And health to all their flesh.—Proverbs 4:20-22

Beloved, I pray that in all respects you may prosper and be in good health, just as your soul prospers.
—3 John 1:2 NASB

HEAR, HELP ME TO

Your ears shall hear a word behind you, saying, "This is the way, walk in it," Whenever you turn to the right hand Or whenever you turn to the left.
—Isaiah 30:21

HEAR MY CRY

Hear my cry, O God; Attend to my prayer. From the end of the earth I will cry to You, When my heart is overwhelmed; Lead me to the rock that is higher than I. For You have been a shelter for me, A strong tower from the enemy.—Psalm 61:1-3

HEARING

In that day the deaf shall hear the words of a book, and out of their gloom and darkness the eyes of the blind shall see.—Isaiah 29:18 RSV

Your ears shall hear a word behind you, saying, "This is the way, walk in it," Whenever you turn to the right hand Or whenever you turn to the left.
—Isaiah 30:21

But blessed are your eyes for they see, and your ears for they hear.—Matthew 13:16

And they were astonished beyond measure, saying, "He has done all things well. He makes both the deaf to hear and the mute to speak."—Mark 7:37

HEART

(See also "Ministry Helps, Heart Disease—Prayer and Counsel for" and "Brokenhearted" Scriptures.)

May He grant you according to your heart's desire, And fulfill all your purpose.—Psalm 20:4

Delight yourself also in the LORD, And He shall give you the desires of your heart. Commit your way to the LORD, Trust also in Him, And He shall bring it to pass.—Psalm 37:4-5

My flesh and my heart fail; But God is the strength of my heart and my portion forever.—Psalm 73:26

Keep your heart with all diligence, For out of it spring the issues of life.—Proverbs 4:23

A sound heart is life to the body, But envy is rottenness to the bones.—Proverbs 14:30

A merry heart makes a cheerful countenance, But by sorrow of the heart the spirit is broken.
—Proverbs 15:13

A merry heart does good, like medicine, But a broken spirit dries the bones.—Proverbs 17:22

Therefore remove sorrow from your heart, And put away evil from your flesh, For childhood and youth are vanity.—Ecclesiastes 11:10

Say to those who are fearful-hearted, "Be strong, do not fear! Behold, your God will come with vengeance, With the recompense of God; He will come and save you."—Isaiah 35:4

"The Spirit of the Lord GOD is upon Me, Because the LORD has anointed Me To preach good tidings to the poor; He has sent Me to heal the broken-hearted, To proclaim liberty to the captives, And the opening of the prison to those who are *bound;*
—Isaiah 61:1

"The Spirit of the LORD is upon Me, Because He has anointed Me To preach the gospel to the *poor; He has sent Me to heal the brokenhearted, To proclaim liberty to* the *captives And recovery of sight to* the *blind, To set at liberty those who are oppressed;*—Luke 4:18

For the hearts of this people have grown dull. Their ears are hard of hearing, And their eyes they have closed, Lest they should see with their *eyes and hear with* their *ears, lest they should understand with* their *hearts and turn, so that I should heal them."*—Acts 28:27

Now hope does not disappoint, because the love of God has been poured out in our hearts by the Holy Spirit who was given to us.—Romans 5:5

For with the heart one believes unto righteousness, and with the mouth confession is made unto salvation.—Romans 10:10

HEAVEN

In My Father's house are many mansions; if it were not so, I would have told you. I go to prepare a place for you. And if I go and pre-pare a place for you, I will come again and receive you to Myself; that where I am, there you may be also.—John 14:2-3

For our citizenship is in heaven, from which we also eagerly wait for the Savior, the Lord Jesus Christ,
                        —Philippians 3:20

For this we say to you by the word of the Lord, that we who are alive and *remain until the coming of the Lord will by no means precede those who are asleep. For the Lord Himself will descend from heaven with a shout, with the voice of an archangel, and with the trumpet of God. And the dead in Christ will rise first. Then we who are alive* and *remain shall be caught up together with them in the clouds to meet the Lord in the air. And thus we shall always be with the Lord. Therefore comfort one another with these words*—1 Thessalonians 4:15-18

They shall neither hunger anymore nor thirst anymore; the sun shall not strike them, nor any heat; for the Lamb who is in the midst of the throne will shepherd them and lead them to living fountains of waters. And God will wipe away every tear from their eyes."—Revelation 7:16-17

HELP

May the LORD answer you in the day of trouble; May the name of the God of Jacob defend you; May He send you help from the sanctuary, And strengthen you out of Zion; May He remember all your offerings, And accept your burnt sacrifice. Se-lah May He grant you according to your heart's de-sire, And fulfill all your purpose.—Psalm 20:1-4

Give us help from trouble, For the help of man is useless. Through God we will do valiantly, For it is He who shall tread down our enemies.
—Psalm 60:11-12

HEMORRHAGE

A woman who had had a hemorrhage for twelve years, and had endured much at the hands of many physicians, and had spent all that she had and was not helped at all, but instead had become worse—after hearing about Jesus, she came up in the crowd behind Him *and touched His cloak. For she had been saying* to herself, *"If I just touch His garments, I will get well." And immediately the flow of her blood was dried up; and she felt in her body that she was healed of her disease. And immediately Jesus, perceiving in Himself that power from Him had gone out, turned around in the crowd and said, "Who touched My garments?" And His disciples said to Him, "You see the crowd pressing in on You, and You say, 'Who touched Me?'" And He looked around to see the woman who had done this. But the woman, fearing and trembling, aware of what had happened to her, came and fell down before Him and told Him the whole truth. And He said to her, "Daughter, your faith has made you well; go in peace and be cured of your disease."*

—Mark 5:25-34 NASB

Now a woman, having a flow of blood for twelve years, who had spent all her livelihood on physicians and could not be healed by any, Now when the woman saw that she was not hidden, she came trembling; and falling down before Him, she declared to Him in the presence of all the people the reason she had touched Him and how she was healed immediately.—Luke 8:43,47

HOLINESS

But now having been set free from sin, and having become slaves of God, you have your fruit to holiness, and the end, everlasting life.—Romans 6:22

Therefore, having these promises, beloved, let us cleanse ourselves from all filthiness of the flesh and spirit, perfecting holiness in the fear of God.
—2 Corinthians 7:1

just as He chose us in Him before the foundation of the world, that we should be holy and without blame before Him in love, having predestined us to adoption as sons by Jesus Christ to Himself, ac-cording to the good pleasure of His will,—Ephesians 1:4-5

For God did not call us to uncleanness, but in holiness.—1 Thessalonians 4:7

Now may the God of peace Himself sanctify you completely; and may your whole spirit, soul, and body be preserved blameless at the coming of our Lord Jesus Christ.—1 Thessalonians 5:23

but as He who called you is *holy, you also be holy in all* your *conduct, because it is written, "Be holy, for I am holy."*—1 Peter 1:15-16

HOLY SPIRIT

If you then, being evil, know how to give good gifts to your children, how much more will your *heavenly Father give the Holy Spirit to those who ask Him!*—Luke 11:13

And I will pray the Father, and He will give you another Helper, that He may abide with you forever—the Spirit of truth, whom the world cannot receive, because it neither sees Him nor knows Him; but you know Him, for He dwells with you and will be in you.—John 14:16-17

And when He had said this, He breathed on them, *and said to them, "Receive the Holy Spirit.*
*—*John 20:22

But you shall receive power when the Holy Spirit has come upon you; and you shall be witnesses to Me in Jerusalem, and in all Judea and Samaria, and to the end of the earth.”—Acts 1:8

HOPE

I have set the LORD always before me; Because He is at my right hand I shall not be moved. Therefore my heart is glad, and my glory rejoices; My flesh also will rest in hope.—Psalm 16:8-9

Be of good courage, And He shall strengthen your heart, All you who hope in the LORD.
—Psalm 31:24

Why are you cast down, O my soul? And why are you disquieted within me? Hope in God, for I shall yet praise Him For the help of His countenance. O my God, my soul is cast down within me; Therefore I will remember You from the land of the Jordan, …—Psalm 42:5-6

The LORD takes pleasure in those who fear Him, In those who hope in His mercy.—Psalm 147:11

This I recall to my mind, Therefore I have hope. Through the LORD's mercies we are not consumed, Because His compassions fail not. The LORD is good to those who wait for Him, To the soul who seeks Him.—Lamentations 3:21-22,25

Therefore I will look to the LORD; I will wait for the God of my salvation; My God will hear me. —Micah 7:7

Therefore my heart rejoiced, and my tongue was glad; Moreover my flesh also will rest in hope. For You will not leave my soul in Hades, Nor will You allow Your Holy One to see corruption.—Acts 2:26-27

For whatever things were written before were written for our learning, that we through the patience and comfort of the Scriptures might have hope. —Romans 15:4

Now may the God of hope fill you with all joy and peace in believing, that you may abound in hope by the power of the Holy Spirit.—Romans 15:13

To them God willed to make known what are the riches of the glory of this mystery among the Gentiles: which is Christ in you, the hope of glory. —Colossians 1:27

This is *a faithful saying and worthy of all acceptance. For to this* end *we both labor and suffer reproach, because we trust in the living God, who is* the *Savior of all men, especially of those who believe.*—1 Timothy 4:9-10

Thus God, determining to show more abundantly to the heirs of promise the immutability of His counsel, confirmed it *by an oath, that by two immutable things, in which it* is *impossible for God to lie, we might have strong consolation, who have fled for refuge to lay hold of the hope set before* us.

—Hebrews 6:17-18

Therefore gird up the loins of your mind, be sober, and rest your *hope fully upon the grace that is to be brought to you at the revelation of Jesus Christ;*

—1 Peter 1:13

not by works of righteousness which we have done, but according to His mercy He saved us, through the washing of regeneration and renewing of the Holy Spirit, whom He poured out on us abundantly through Jesus Christ our Savior, that having been justified by His grace we should become heirs according to the hope of eternal life.—Titus 3:5-7

And everyone who has this hope in Him purifies himself, just as He is pure.—1 John 3:3

HUNGER

They shall neither hunger anymore nor thirst anymore; the sun shall not strike them, nor any heat; "for the Lamb who is in the midst of the throne will shepherd them and lead them to living fountains of waters. And God will wipe away every tear from their eyes."—Revelation 7:16-17

IDENTITY

For the LORD will not forsake His people, for His great name's sake, because it has pleased the LORD to make you His people.—1 Samuel 12:22

Oh come, let us worship and bow down; Let us kneel before the LORD our Maker. For He is our God, And we are the people of His pasture, And the sheep of His hand. Today, if you will hear His voice:—Psalm 95:6-7

Know that the LORD, He is God; It is He who has made us, and not we ourselves; We are His people and the sheep of His pasture.
          —Psalm 100:3

For You formed my inward parts; You covered me in my mother's womb. I will praise You, for I am fearfully and wonderfully made; Marvelous are Your works, And that my soul knows very well.
—Psalm 139:13-14

But now, thus says the LORD, who created you, O Jacob, And He who formed you, O Israel: "Fear not, for I have redeemed you; I have called you by your name; You are Mine.—Isaiah 43:1

For I will pour water on him who is thirsty, And floods on the dry ground; I will pour My Spirit on your descendants, And My blessing on your offspring;—Isaiah 44:3

"Can a woman forget her nursing child, And not have compassion on the son of her womb? Surely they may forget, Yet I will not forget you. See, I have inscribed you on the palms of My hands; Your walls are continually before Me.—Isaiah 49:15-16

You did not choose Me, but I chose you and appointed you that you should go and bear fruit, and that your fruit should remain, that whatever you ask the Father in My name He may give you.
—John 15:16

having predestined us to adoption as sons by Jesus Christ to Himself, according to the good pleasure of His will, to the praise of the glory of His grace, by which He has made us accepted in the Beloved.
—Ephesians 1:5-6

In Him you also trusted, *after you heard the word of truth, the gospel of your salvation; in whom also, having believed, you were sealed with the Holy Spirit of promise,*—Ephesians 1:13

For we are His workmanship, created in Christ Jesus for good works, which God prepared beforehand that we should walk in them.—Ephesians 2:10

Therefore, as the *elect of God, holy and beloved, put on tender mercies, kindness, humility, meekness, longsuffering;*—Colossians 3:12

But you are *a chosen generation, a royal priesthood, a holy nation, His own special people, that you may proclaim the praises of Him who called you out of darkness into His marvelous light;*—1 Peter 2:9

Behold what manner of love the Father has bestowed on us, that we should be called children of God! Therefore the world does not know us, because it did not know Him. Beloved, now we are children of God; and it has not yet been revealed what we shall be, but we know that when He is revealed, we shall be like Him, for we shall see Him as He is.
—1 John 3:1-2

INFIRMITIES

And Jesus went about all Galilee, teaching in their synagogues, preaching the gospel of the kingdom, and healing all kinds of sickness and all kinds of disease among the people.—Matthew 4:23

Then His fame went throughout all Syria; and they brought to Him all sick people who were afflicted with various diseases and torments, and those who were demon-possessed, epileptics, and paralytics; and He healed them.—Matthew 4:24

When evening had come, they brought to Him many who were demon-possessed. And He cast out the spirits with a word, and healed all who were sick, that it might be fulfilled which was spoken by Isaiah the prophet, saying: "He Himself took our infirmities And bore our sicknesses."

—Matthew 8:16-17

Then Jesus went about all the cities and villages, teaching in their synagogues, preaching the gospel of the kingdom, and healing every sickness and every disease among the people.—Matthew 9:35

And when He had called His twelve disciples to Him, He gave them power over unclean spirits, to cast them out, and to heal all kinds of sickness and all kinds of disease.—Matthew 10:1

Heal the sick, cleanse the lepers, raise the dead, cast out demons. Freely you have received, freely give.
—Matthew 10:8

And when Jesus went out He saw a great multitude; and He was moved with compassion for them, and healed their sick.—Matthew 14:14

Then He healed many who were sick with various diseases, and cast out many demons; and He did not allow the demons to speak, because they knew Him.—Mark 1:34

and to have power to heal sicknesses and to cast out demons:—Mark 3:15

And they cast out many demons, and anointed with oil many who were sick, and healed them.
—Mark 6:13

When the sun was setting, all those who had any that were sick with various diseases brought them to Him; and He laid His hands on every one of them and healed them.—Luke 4:40

However, the report went around concerning Him all the more; and great multitudes came together to hear, and to be healed by Him of their infirmities.
—Luke 5:15

So when he heard about Jesus, he sent elders of the Jews to Him, pleading with Him to come and heal his servant. Therefore I did not even think myself worthy to come to You. But say the word, and my servant will be healed. And those who were sent, returning to the house, found the servant well who had been sick.—Luke 7:3,7,10

and certain women who had been healed of evil spirits and infirmities—Mary called Magdalene, out of whom had come seven demons,—Luke 8:2

He sent them to preach the kingdom of God and to heal the sick.—Luke 9:2

And heal the sick there, and say to them, 'The kingdom of God has come near to you.'—Luke 10:9

Also a multitude gathered from the surrounding cities to Jerusalem, bringing sick people and those who were tormented by unclean spirits, and they were all healed.—Acts 5:16

So when this was done, the rest of those on the island who had diseases also came and were healed.
—Acts 28:9

Is anyone among you suffering? Let him pray. Is anyone cheerful? Let him sing psalms. Is anyone among you sick? Let him call for the elders of the church, and let them pray over him, anointing him with oil in the name of the Lord. And the prayer of faith will save the sick, and the Lord will raise him up. And if he has committed sins, he will be forgiven. Confess your trespasses to one another, and pray for one another, that you may be healed. The effective, fervent prayer of a righteous man avails much.—James 5:13-16

INFLAMMATION

My wounds are foul and *festering Because of my foolishness. I am troubled, I am bowed down greatly; I go mourning all the day long. For my loins are full of inflammation, and* there is *no soundness in my flesh. I am feeble and severely broken; I groan because of the turmoil of my heart. For in You, O LORD, I hope; You will hear, O Lord my God.*
—Psalm 38:5-8,15

INTEGRITY

I know also, my God, that You test the heart and have pleasure in uprightness. As for me, in the uprightness of my heart I have willingly offered all these things; and now with joy I have seen Your people, who are present here to offer willingly to You.
—1 Chronicles 29:17

He who walks uprightly, And works righteousness, And speaks the truth in his heart; He who does not put out his money at usury, Nor does he take a bribe against the innocent. He who does these things shall never be moved.—Psalm 15:2,5

Who is the man who desires life, And loves many days, that he may see good? Keep your tongue from evil, And your lips from speaking deceit.
Psalm 34:12-13

As for me, You uphold me in my integrity, And set me before Your face forever.—Psalm 41:12

Behold, You desire truth in the inward parts, And in the hidden part You will make me to know wisdom.—Psalm 51:6

He who walks with integrity walks securely, But he who perverts his ways will become known.
—Proverbs 10:9

The integrity of the upright will guide them, But the perversity of the unfaithful will destroy them.
—Proverbs 11:3

A righteous man *hates lying, But a wicked* man *is loathsome and comes to shame.*—Proverbs 13:5

He who walks righteously and speaks uprightly, He who despises the gain of oppressions, Who gestures with his hands, refusing bribes, Who stops his ears from hearing of bloodshed, And shuts his eyes from seeing evil: He will dwell on high; His place of defense will be *the fortress of rocks; Bread will be given him, His water* will be *sure.*
—Isaiah 33:15-16

does not rejoice in iniquity, but rejoices in the truth;
—1 Corinthians 13:6

INVALID

But the one who was healed did not know who it was, for Jesus had withdrawn, a multitude being in that place.—John 5:13

JOINTS

from whom the whole body, joined and knit together by what every joint supplies, according to the effective working by which every part does its share, causes growth of the body for the edifying of itself in love.
—Ephesians 4:16

and not holding fast to the Head, from whom all the body, nourished and knit together by joints and ligaments, grows with the increase that is from God.—Colossians 2:19

JOY

Then he said to them, "Go your way, eat the fat, drink the sweet, and send portions to those for whom nothing is prepared; for this day is holy to our Lord. Do not sorrow, for the joy of the LORD is your strength."—Nehemiah 8:10

He will yet fill your mouth with laughing, And your lips with rejoicing.—Job 8:21

For You, LORD, have made me glad through Your work; I will triumph in the works of Your hands.
—Psalm 92:4

Those who sow in tears Shall reap in joy.
—Psalm 126:5

If you keep My commandments, you will abide in My love, just as I have kept My Father's commandments and abide in His love. "These things I have spoken to you, that My joy may remain in you, and that *your joy may be full.*—John 15:10-11

Until now you have asked nothing in My name. Ask, and you will receive, that your joy may be full.—John 16:24

Therefore my heart rejoiced, and my tongue was glad; Moreover my flesh also will rest in hope. For You will not leave my soul in Hades, Nor will You allow Your Holy One to see corruption. You have made known to me the ways of life; You will make me full of joy in Your presence.'—Acts 2:26-28

You have loved righteousness and hated lawlessness; Therefore God, Your God, has anointed You With the oil of gladness more than Your companions."
—Hebrews 1:9

whom having not seen you love. Though now you do not see Him, *yet believing, you rejoice with joy inexpressible and full of glory, receiving the end of your faith—the salvation of* your *souls.*
—1 Peter 1:8-9

My brethren, count it all joy when you fall into various trials, knowing that the testing of your faith produces patience.—James 1:2-3

JUSTICE

I know that the LORD will maintain The cause of the afflicted, And justice for the poor. Surely the righteous shall give thanks to Your name; The upright shall dwell in Your presence.
—Psalm 140:12-13

KNEES

Strengthen the weak hands, And make firm the feeble knees. Say to those who are *fearful-hearted, "Be strong, do not fear! Behold, your God will come* with *vengeance,* With *the recompense of God; He will come and save you."*—Isaiah 35:3-4

Therefore strengthen the hands which hang down, and the feeble knees, and make straight paths for your feet, so that what is lame may not be dislocated, but rather be healed.—Hebrews 12:12-13

LAME

Behold, at that time I will deal with all who afflict you; I will save the lame, And gather those who were driven out; I will appoint them for praise and fame In every land where they were put to shame.
—Zephaniah 3:19

But for you who fear my name the sun of righteousness shall rise, with healing in its wings. You shall go forth leaping like calves from the stall.
—Malachi 4:2 RSV

Then great multitudes came to Him, having with them the *lame, blind, mute, maimed, and many others; and they laid them down at Jesus' feet, and He healed them.*—Matthew 15:30

Then the *blind and* the *lame came to Him in the temple, and He healed them.*—Matthew 21:14

Now as the lame man who was healed held on to Peter and John, all the people ran together to them in the porch which is called Solomon's, greatly amazed.—Acts 3:11

And Peter said to him, "Aeneas, Jesus the Christ heals you. Arise and make your bed." Then he arose immediately.—Acts 9:34

... a certain man without strength in his feet was sitting, a cripple from his mother's womb, who had never walked. This *man heard Paul speaking. Paul, observing him intently and seeing that he had faith to be healed, said with a loud voice, "Stand up straight on your feet!" And he leaped and walked.*—Acts 14:8-10

and make straight paths for your feet, so that what is lame may not be dislocated, but rather be healed.
—Hebrews 12:13

LEPROSY/SKIN DISEASES

So Moses cried out to the LORD, saying, "Please heal her, O God, I pray!"—Numbers 12:13

Then he brought the letter to the king of Israel, which said, Now be advised, when this letter comes to you, that I have sent Naaman my servant to you, that you may heal him of his leprosy. And it happened, when the king of Israel read the letter, that he tore his clothes and said, "Am I God, to kill and make alive, that this man sends a man to me to heal him of his leprosy? Therefore please consider, and see how he seeks a quarrel with me." But Naaman became furious, and went away and said, "Indeed, I said to myself, 'He will surely come out to me, and stand and call on the name of the LORD his God, and wave his hand over the place, and heal the leprosy.'"—2 Kings 5:6-7,11

And behold, a leper came and worshiped Him, saying, "Lord, if You are willing, You can make me clean." Then Jesus put out His hand and touched him, saying, "I am willing; be cleansed." Immediately his leprosy was cleansed.—Matthew 8:2-3

Heal the sick, cleanse the lepers, raise the dead, cast out demons. Freely you have received, freely give.
—Matthew 10:8

LIFE AND EXTENDED LIFE

So you shall serve the LORD your God, and He will bless your bread and your water. And I will take sickness away from the midst of you. No one shall suffer miscarriage or be barren in your land; I will fulfill the number of your days.
—Exodus 23:25-26

And the LORD your God will circumcise your heart and the heart of your descendants, to love the LORD your God with all your heart and with all your soul, that you may live.—Deuteronomy 30:6

And may he be to you a restorer of life and a nourisher of your old age; for your daughter-in-law, who loves you, who is better to you than seven sons, has borne him.—Ruth 4:15

And he said to his father, "My head, my head!" So he said to a servant, "Carry him to his mother." When Elisha came into the house, there was the child, lying dead on his bed. He went in therefore, shut the door behind the two of them, and prayed to the LORD. *And he went up and lay on the child, and put his mouth on his mouth, his eyes on his eyes, and his hands on his hands; and he stretched himself out on the child, and the flesh of the child became warm. He returned and walked back and forth in the house, and again went up and stretched himself out on him; then the child sneezed seven times, and the child opened his eyes.*—2 Kings 4:19,32-35

The Spirit of God has made me, And the breath of the Almighty gives me life.—Job 33:4

He asked life from You, and *You gave* it *to him— Length of days forever and ever.*—Psalm 21:4

The LORD *will preserve him and keep him alive, And he will be blessed on the earth; You will not deliver him to the will of his enemies. The* LORD *will strengthen him on his bed of illness; You will sustain him on his sickbed.*—Psalm 41:2-3

For You have delivered my soul from death. Have You not kept my feet from falling, That I may walk before God In the light of the living?
—Psalm 56:13

He will spare the poor and needy, And will save the souls of the needy.—Psalm 72:13

Let the groaning of the prisoner come before You; According to the greatness of Your power Preserve those who are appointed to die;—Psalm 79:11

He weakened my strength in the way; He shortened my days. I said, "O my God, Do not take me away in the midst of my days; Your years are throughout all generations.—Psalm 102:23-24

Who forgives all your iniquities, Who heals all your diseases, Who redeems your life from destruction, Who crowns you with lovingkindness and tender mercies, Who satisfies your mouth with good things, So that your youth is renewed like the eagle's.
—Psalm 103:3-5

Their soul abhorred all manner of food, And they drew near to the gates of death. Then they cried out to the LORD *in their trouble,* And *He saved them out of their distresses. He sent His word and healed them, And delivered* them *from their destructions.*—Psalm 107:18-20

I love the LORD, *because He has heard My voice and my supplications. Because He has inclined His ear to me, Therefore I will call upon Him as long as I live. The pains of death surrounded me, And the pangs of Sheol laid hold of me; I found trouble and sorrow. Then I called upon the name of the* LORD: *"O* LORD, *I implore You, deliver my soul!" Gracious is the* LORD, *and righteous; Yes, our God is merciful. The* LORD *preserves the simple; I was brought low, and He saved me. Return to your rest, O my soul, For the* LORD *has dealt bountifully with you. For You have delivered my soul from death, My eyes from tears, And my feet from falling. I will walk before the* LORD *In the land of the living.*—Psalm 116:1-9

I shall not die, but live, And declare the works of the LORD. *The* LORD *has chastened me severely, But He has not given me over to death.*
—Psalm 118:17-18

Uphold me according to Your word, that I may live; And do not let me be ashamed of my hope. Hold me up, and I shall be safe, And I shall observe Your statutes continually. Plead my cause and redeem me; Revive me according to Your word.
—Psalm 119:116-117,154

My son, do not forget my law, But let your heart keep my commands; For length of days and long life And peace they will add to you.—Proverbs 3:1-2

My son, let them not depart from your eyes—Keep sound wisdom and discretion; So they will be life to your soul And grace to your neck. Then you will walk safely in your way, And your foot will not stumble.—Proverbs 3:21-23

My son, give attention to my words; Incline your ear to my sayings. Do not let them depart from your eyes; Keep them in the midst of your heart; for they are life to those who find them, And health to all their flesh.—Proverbs 4:20-22

For whoever finds Me finds life, And obtains favor from the LORD.—Proverbs 8:35

He who guards his mouth preserves his life, But he who opens wide his lips shall have destruction.
—Proverbs 13:3

Death and life are *in the power of the tongue, And those who love it will eat its fruit.*
—Proverbs 18:21

… Thus says the LORD, *the God of David your father: "I have heard your prayer, I have seen your tears; surely I will add to your days fifteen years.*
—Isaiah 38:5

115

"Therefore I say to you, do not worry about your life, what you will eat or what you will drink; nor about your body, what you will put on. Is not life more than food and the body more than clothing?
—Matthew 6:25

For God so loved the world that He gave His only begotten Son, that whoever believes in Him should not perish but have everlasting life.—John 3:16

Most assuredly, I say to you, he who believes in Me has everlasting life.—John 6:47

It is the Spirit who gives life; the flesh profits nothing. The words that I speak to you are spirit, and they are life.—John 6:63

The thief does not come except to steal, and to kill, and to destroy. I have come that they may have life, and that they may have it more abundantly.
—John 10:10

When Jesus heard that, He said, "This sickness is not unto death, but for the glory of God, that the Son of God may be glorified through it."
—John 11:4

Jesus said to her, "I am the resurrection and the life. He who believes in Me, though he may die, he shall live. "And whoever lives and believes in Me shall never die. Do you believe this?"—John 11:25-26

116

But if the Spirit of Him who raised Jesus from the dead dwells in you, He who raised Christ from the dead will also give life to your mortal bodies through His Spirit who dwells in you.—Romans 8:11

yet for us there is *one God, the Father, of whom* are *all things, and we for Him; and one Lord Jesus Christ, through whom* are *all things, and through whom we* live.—1 Corinthians 8:6

I have been crucified with Christ; it is no longer I who live, but Christ lives in me; and the life *which I now live in the flesh I live by faith in the Son of God, who loved me and gave Himself for me.*
—Galatians 2:20

For indeed he was sick almost unto death; but God had mercy on him, and not only on him but on me also, lest I should have sorrow upon sorrow.
—Philippians 2:27

If then you were raised with Christ, seek those things which are above, where Christ is, sitting at the right hand of God. Set your mind on things above, not on things on the earth. For you died, and your life is hidden with Christ in God. When Christ who is *our life appears, then you also will appear with Him in glory.*—Colossians 3:1-4

For bodily exercise profits a little, but godliness is profitable for all things, having promise of the life that now is and of that which is to come.
—1 Timothy 4:8

Blessed is the man who endures temptation; for when he has been approved, he will receive the crown of life which the Lord has promised to those who love Him.—James 1:12

We know that we have passed from death to life, because we love the brethren. He who does not love his *brother abides in death. Whoever hates his brother is a murderer, and you know that no murderer has eternal life abiding in him.*
—1 John 3:14-15

LOVE

Love suffers long and *is kind; love does not envy; love does not parade itself, is not puffed up; does not behave rudely, does not seek its own, is not provoked, thinks no evil; does not rejoice in iniquity, but rejoices in the truth; bears all things, believes all things, hopes all things, endures all things. Love never fails.* …—1 Corinthians 13:4-8

But the fruit of the Spirit is love, joy, peace, longsuffering, kindness, goodness, faithfulness,
—Galatians 5:22

And this I pray, that your love may abound still more and more in knowledge and all discernment,
—Philippians 1:9

Beloved, let us love one another, for love is of God; and everyone who loves is born of God and knows God. He who does not love does not know God, for God is love. In this the love of God was manifested toward us, that God has sent His only begotten Son into the world, that we might live through Him. In this is love, not that we loved God, but that He loved us and sent His Son to be *the propitiation for our sins. Beloved, if God so loved us, we also ought to love one another. No one has seen God at any time. If we love one another, God abides in us, and His love has been perfected in us. By this we know that we abide in Him, and He in us, because He has given us of His Spirit. And we have seen and testify that the Father has sent the Son* as *Savior of the world. Whoever confesses that Jesus is the Son of God, God abides in him, and he in God. And we have known and believed the love that God has for us. God is love, and he who abides in love abides in God, and God in him. Love has been perfected among us in this: that we may have boldness in the day of judgment; because as He is, so are we in this world. There is no fear in love; but perfect love casts out fear, because fear involves torment. But he who fears has not been made perfect in love. We love Him because He first loved us. If someone says, "I love God," and hates his brother, he is a liar; for he who does not love his brother whom he has seen, how can he love God whom he has not seen? And this commandment we have from Him: that he who loves God* must *love his brother also.*—1 John 4:7-21

Mercy, peace, and love be multiplied to you.
—Jude 1:2

LOVE GOD

in that I command you today to love the LORD *your God, to walk in His ways, and to keep His commandments, His statutes, and His judgments, that you may live and multiply; and the* LORD *your God will bless you in the land which you go to possess.*
—Deuteronomy 30:16

And we know that all things work together for good to those who love God, to those who are the called according to His *purpose.*—Romans 8:28

But as it is written: "Eye has not seen, nor ear heard, Nor have entered into the heart of man The things which God has prepared for those who love Him."—1 Corinthians 2:9

LOVE, GOD'S

But the mercy of the LORD is from everlasting to everlasting On those who fear Him, And His righteousness to children's children,—Psalm 103:17

The LORD is near to all who call upon Him, To all who call upon Him in truth.—Psalm 145:18

The LORD has appeared of old to me, saying: *"Yes, I have loved you with an everlasting love; Therefore with lovingkindness I have drawn you.*
—Jeremiah 31:3

"I will betroth you to Me forever; Yes, I will betroth you to Me In righteousness and justice, In lovingkindness and mercy; I will betroth you to Me in faithfulness, And you shall know the LORD.
—Hosea 2:19-20

for the Father Himself loves you, because you have loved Me, and have believed that I came forth from God.—John 16:27

Now hope does not disappoint, because the love of God has been poured out in our hearts by the Holy Spirit who was given to us.—Romans 5:5

But God, who is rich in mercy, because of His great love with which He loved us, even when we were dead in trespasses, made us alive together with Christ (by grace you have been saved),—Ephesians 2:4-5

121

But whoever keeps His word, truly the love of God is perfected in him. By this we know that we are in Him.—1 John 2:5

In this is love, not that we loved God, but that He loved us and sent His Son to be *the propitiation for our sins.*—1 John 4:10

LOVE OTHERS

He who covers a transgression seeks love, But he who repeats a matter separates friends.
—Proverbs 17:9

But I say to you, love your enemies, bless those who curse you, do good to those who hate you, and pray for those who spitefully use you and persecute you, that you may be sons of your Father in heaven; for He makes His sun rise on the evil and on the good, and sends rain on the just and on the unjust.
—Matthew 5:44-45

A new commandment I give to you, that you love one another; as I have loved you, that you also love one another. By this all will know that you are My disciples, if you have love for one another."
—John 13:34-35

Let nothing be done through selfish ambition or conceit, but in lowliness of mind let each esteem others better than himself. Let each of you look out not only for his own interests, but also for the interests of others.—Philippians 2:3-4

Therefore, as the *elect of God, holy and beloved, put on tender mercies, kindness, humility, meekness, longsuffering; bearing with one another, and forgiving one another, if anyone has a complaint against another; even as Christ forgave you, so you also* must do. *But above all these things put on love, which is the bond of perfection.*—Colossians 3:12-14

And above all things have fervent love for one another, for "love will cover a multitude of sins.
—1 Peter 4:8

If you really fulfill the *royal law according to the Scripture, "You shall love your neighbor as yourself," you do well;*—James 2:8

He who loves his brother abides in the light, and there is no cause for stumbling in him.
—1 John 2:10

Beloved, let us love one another, for love is of God; and everyone who loves is born of God and knows God.—1 John 4:7

No one has seen God at any time. If we love one another, God abides in us, and His love has been perfected in us.—1 John 4:12

We love Him because He first loved us.
—1 John 4:19

LUNGS (SEE BREATH)

MAIMED

Then great multitudes came to Him, having with them the lame, blind, mute, maimed, and many others; and they laid them down at Jesus' feet, and He healed them.—Matthew 15:30

MERCY

(for the LORD your God is a merciful God), He will not forsake you nor destroy you, nor forget the covenant of your fathers which He swore to them.
—Deuteronomy 4:31

Behold, the eye of the LORD is on those who fear Him, On those who hope in His mercy,
—Psalm 33:18

For the LORD is good; His mercy is everlasting, And His truth endures to all generations.
—Psalm 100:5

The LORD takes pleasure in those who fear Him, In those who hope in His mercy.—Psalm 147:11

Therefore the LORD will wait, that He may be gracious to you; And therefore He will be exalted, that He may have mercy on you. For the LORD is a God of justice; Blessed are all those who wait for Him.—Isaiah 30:18

Seek the LORD while He may be found, Call upon Him while He is near. Let the wicked forsake his way, And the unrighteous man his thoughts; Let him return to the LORD, And He will have mercy on him; And to our God, For He will abundantly pardon.—Isaiah 55:6-7

"I will betroth you to Me forever; Yes, I will betroth you to Me In righteousness and justice, In lovingkindness and mercy;—Hosea 2:19

Who is a God like You, Pardoning iniquity And passing over the transgression of the remnant of His heritage? He does not retain His anger forever, Because He delights in mercy.—Micah 7:18

not by works of righteousness which we have done, but according to His mercy He saved us, through the washing of regeneration and renewing of the Holy Spirit,—Titus 3:5

Mercy, peace, and love be multiplied to you.
—Jude 1:2

MINISTRY

So shall My word be that goes forth from My mouth; It shall not return to Me void, But it shall accomplish what I please, And it shall prosper in the thing for which I sent it.—Isaiah 55:11

They shall not labor in vain, …—Isaiah 65:23

"I am the vine, you are the branches. He who abides in Me, and I in him, bears much fruit; for without Me you can do nothing.—John 15:5

And He said to them, "Go into all the world and preach the gospel to every creature. He who believes and is baptized will be saved; but he who does not believe will be condemned. And these signs will follow those who believe: In My name they will cast out demons; they will speak with new tongues; they will take up serpents; and if they drink anything deadly, it will by no means hurt them; they will lay hands on the sick, and they will recover."—Mark 16:15-18

MOURNING

Hear, O LORD, and have mercy on me; LORD, be my helper!" You have turned for me my mourning into dancing; You have put off my sackcloth and clothed me with gladness,—Psalm 30:10-11

Your sun shall no longer go down, Nor shall your moon withdraw itself; For the LORD will be your everlasting light, And the days of your mourning shall be ended.—Isaiah 60:20

MOUTH

Now therefore, go, and I will be with your mouth and teach you what you shall say."—Exodus 4:12

There is one who speaks like the piercings of a sword, But the tongue of the wise promotes *health. The truthful lip shall be established forever, But a lying tongue* is *but for a moment.*

—Proverbs 12:18-19

Death and life are *in the power of the tongue, And those who love it will eat its fruit.*

—Proverbs 18:21

"The Lord God has given Me The tongue of the learned, That I should know how to speak A word in season to him who is weary. He awakens Me morning by morning, He awakens My ear To hear as the learned.—Isaiah 50:4

So shall My word be that goes forth from My mouth; It shall not return to Me void, But it shall accomplish what I please, And it shall prosper in the thing *for which I sent it.*—Isaiah 55:11

that if you confess with your mouth the Lord Jesus and believe in your heart that God has raised Him from the dead, you will be saved. For with the heart one believes unto righteousness, and with the mouth confession is made unto salvation.

—Romans 10:9-10

MUSCLES

For You formed my inward parts; You covered me in my mother's womb. I will praise You, for I am fearfully and wonderfully made; Marvelous are Your works, And that my soul knows very well.

—Psalm 139:13-14

I will put sinews on you and bring flesh upon you, cover you with skin and put breath in you; and you shall live. Then you shall know that I am the LORD. """—Ezekiel 37:6

MUTE

Now therefore, go, and I will be with your mouth and teach you what you shall say." ... Now you shall speak to him and put the words in his mouth. And I will be with your mouth and with his mouth, and I will teach you what you shall do.

—Exodus 4:12,15

But the LORD *said to me: " … For you shall go to all to whom I send you, And whatever I command you, you shall speak.*—Jeremiah 1:7

Then the LORD *put forth His hand and touched my mouth, and the* LORD *said to me: "Behold, I have put My words in your mouth.*—Jeremiah 1:9

Then one was brought to Him who was demon- possessed, blind and mute; and He healed him, so that the blind and mute man both spoke and saw.
—Matthew 12:22

Then great multitudes came to Him, having with them the *lame, blind, mute, maimed, and many others; and they laid them down at Jesus' feet, and He healed them.*—Matthew 15:30

And they were astonished beyond measure, saying, "He has done all things well. He makes both the deaf to hear and the mute to speak."—Mark 7:37

NEEDS

The LORD *is my shepherd; I shall not want.*
—Psalm 23:1

For the LORD *God* is *a sun and shield; The* LORD *will give grace and glory; No good* thing *will He withhold From those who walk uprightly.*
—Psalm 84:11

I will abundantly bless her provision; I will satisfy her poor with bread.—Psalm 132:15

But seek first the kingdom of God and His righteousness, and all these things shall be added to you.—Matthew 6:33

If you then, being evil, know how to give good gifts to your children, how much more will your Father who is in heaven give good things to those who ask Him!—Matthew 7:11

"Most assuredly, I say to you, he who believes in Me, the works that I do he will do also; and greater works *than these he will do, because I go to My Father. And whatever you ask in My name, that I will do, that the Father may be glorified in the Son. If you ask anything in My name, I will do* it.
—John 14:12-14

And we know that all things work together for good to those who love God, to those who are the called according to His *purpose.*—Romans 8:28

And God is able to make all grace abound toward you, that you, always having all sufficiency in all things, may have an abundance for every good work.—2 Corinthians 9:8

I can do all things through Christ who strengthens me.—Philippians 4:13

And my God shall supply all your need according to His riches in glory by Christ Jesus.
—Philippians 4:19

as His divine power has given to us all things that pertain *to life and godliness, through the knowledge of Him who called us by glory and virtue,*
—2 Peter 1:3

NOSES

And the LORD *God formed man* of *the dust of the ground, and breathed into his nostrils the breath of life; and man became a living being.*—Genesis 2:7

As long as my breath is *in me, And the breath of God in my nostrils,*—Job 27:3

He returned and walked back and forth in the house, and again went up and stretched himself out on him; then the child sneezed seven times, and the child opened his eyes.—2 Kings 4:35

OLD AGE

And may he be to you a restorer of life and a nourisher of your old age; for your daughter-in-law, who loves you, who is better to you than seven sons, has borne him."—Ruth 4:15

No one shall suffer miscarriage or be barren in your land; I will fulfill the number of your days.
—Exodus 23:26

OPPRESSION

"The Spirit of the LORD is upon Me, Because He has anointed Me To preach the gospel to the poor; He has sent Me to heal the brokenhearted, To proclaim liberty to the captives And recovery of sight to the blind, To set at liberty those who are oppressed.—Luke 4:18

PAIN

But I am afflicted and in pain; let thy salvation, O God, set me on high!—Psalm 69:29 RSV

News about Him spread all over Syria, and people brought to Him all who were ill with various diseases, those suffering severe pain, the demon-possessed, those having seizures, and the paralyzed, and He healed them.—Matthew 4:24 NIV

And God will wipe away every tear from their eyes; there shall be no more death, nor sorrow, nor crying. There shall be no more pain, for the former things have passed away."—Revelation 21:4

PARALYSIS

*And Jesus said to him, "I will come and heal him."
The centurion answered and said, "Lord, I am not
worthy that You should come under my roof. But
only speak a word, and my servant will be healed.
Then Jesus said to the centurion, "Go your way; and
as you have believed, so let it be done for you." And
his servant was healed that same hour.*

—Matthew 8:7-8,13

*Then His fame went throughout all Syria; and they
brought to Him all sick people who were afflicted
with various diseases and torments, and those who
were demon-possessed, epileptics, and paralytics; and
He healed them.*—Matthew 4:24

*Then behold, they brought to Him a paralytic lying
on a bed. When Jesus saw their faith, He said to the
paralytic, "Son, be of good cheer; your sins are forgiven you." For which is easier to say, 'Your sins
are forgiven you,' or to say, 'Arise and walk'? But
that you may know that the Son of Man has power
on earth to forgive sins"—then He said to the paralytic, "Arise, take up your bed, and go to your
house." And he arose and departed to his house.*

—Matthew 9:2,5-7

PATIENCE

Wait on the LORD; *Be of good courage, And He shall strengthen your heart; Wait, I say, on the* LORD!—*Psalm 27:14*

Rest in the LORD, *and wait patiently for Him; Do not fret because of him who prospers in his way, Because of the man who brings wicked schemes to pass.*—Psalm 37:7

I waited patiently for the LORD; *And He inclined to me, And heard my cry. He also brought me up out of a horrible pit, Out of the miry clay, And set my feet upon a rock,* And *established my steps.*
—Psalm 40:1-2

He who is *slow to wrath has great understanding, But* he who is *impulsive exalts folly.*
—Proverbs 14:29

The discretion of a man makes him slow to anger, And his glory is *to overlook a transgression.*
—Proverbs 19:11

But those who wait on the LORD *Shall renew* their *strength; They shall mount up with wings like eagles, They shall run and not be weary, They shall walk and not faint.*—Isaiah 40:31

rejoicing in hope, patient in tribulation, continuing steadfastly in prayer;—Romans 12:12

Therefore be patient, brethren, until the coming of the Lord. See how the farmer waits for the precious fruit of the earth, waiting patiently for it until it receives the early and latter rain. You also be patient. Establish your hearts, for the coming of the Lord is at hand.—James 5:7-8

PEACE

The LORD will give strength to His people; The LORD will bless His people with peace.
—Psalm 29:11

I will hear what God the LORD will speak, For He will speak peace To His people and to His saints; But let them not turn back to folly.—Psalm 85:8

Great peace have those who love Your law, And nothing causes them to stumble.—Psalm 119:165

When a man's ways please the LORD, He makes even his enemies to be at peace with him.
—Proverbs 16:7

You will keep him *in perfect peace,* Whose *mind* is *stayed* on You, *Because he trusts in You.*
—Isaiah 26:3

"For you shall go out with joy, And be led out with peace; The mountains and the hills Shall break forth into singing before you, And all the trees of the field shall clap their *hands.*—Isaiah 55:12

I have seen his ways, and will heal him; I will also lead him, And restore comforts to him And to his mourners. "I create the fruit of the lips: Peace, peace to him who is *far off and to* him who is *near," Says the* LORD, *"And I will heal him."*
—Isaiah 57:18-19

Behold, I will bring it health and healing; I will heal them and reveal to them the abundance of peace and truth.—Jeremiah 33:6

Blessed are *the peacemakers, For they shall be called sons of God.*—Matthew 5:9

Peace I leave with you, My peace I give to you; not as the world gives do I give to you. Let not your heart be troubled, neither let it be afraid.—John 14:27

Therefore, having been justified by faith, we have peace with God through our Lord Jesus Christ,
—Romans 5:1

For to be carnally minded is *death, but to be spiritually minded* is *life and peace.*—Romans 8:6

And the God of peace will crush Satan under your feet shortly. The grace of our Lord Jesus Christ be *with you. Amen.*—Romans 16:20

Finally, brethren, farewell. Become complete. Be of good comfort, be of one mind, live in peace; and the God of love and peace will be with you.
—2 Corinthians 13:11

Be anxious for nothing, but in everything by prayer and supplication, with thanksgiving, let your requests be made known to God; and the peace of God, which surpasses all understanding, will guard your hearts and minds through Christ Jesus.
—Philippians 4:6-7

Now may the God of peace Himself sanctify you completely; and may your whole spirit, soul, and body be preserved blameless at the coming of our Lord Jesus Christ.—1 Thessalonians 5:23

Therefore humble yourselves under the mighty hand of God, that He may exalt you in due time, casting all your care upon Him, for He cares for you.
—1 Peter 5:6-7

Now the fruit of righteousness is sown in peace by those who make peace.—James 3:18

Mercy, peace, and love be multiplied to you.
—Jude 2

PERSEVERANCE

Uphold my steps in Your paths, That my footsteps may not slip.—Psalm 17:5

Cast your burden on the LORD, And He shall sustain you; He shall never permit the righteous to be moved.—Psalm 55:22

137

eternal life to those who by patient continuance in doing good seek for glory, honor, and immortality;
—Romans 2:7

praying always with all prayer and supplication in the Spirit, being watchful to this end with all perseverance and supplication for all the saints—
—Ephesians 6:18

For you have need of endurance, so that after you have done the will of God, you may receive the promise:—Hebrews 10:36

Therefore we also, since we are surrounded by so great a cloud of witnesses, let us lay aside every weight, and the sin which so easily ensnares us, *and let us run with endurance the race that is set before us,*—Hebrews 12:1

My brethren, count it all joy when you fall into various trials, knowing that the testing of your faith produces patience. But let patience have its perfect work, that you may be perfect and complete, lacking nothing.—James 1:2-4

Indeed we count them blessed who endure. You have heard of the perseverance of Job and seen the end intended by *the Lord—that the Lord is very compassionate and merciful.*—James 5:11

Behold, I am coming quickly! Hold fast what you have, that no one may take your crown.
—Revelation 3:11

POISON

they will take up serpents; and if they drink anything deadly, it will by no means hurt them; …
—Mark 16:18

PRAISE

Blessed be *the* LORD, *Because He has heard the voice of my supplications!*—Psalm 28:6

You have turned for me my mourning into dancing; You have put off my sackcloth and clothed me with gladness, To the end that my *glory may sing praise to You and not be silent. O* LORD *my God, I will give thanks to You forever.*—Psalm 30:11-12

According to Your name, O God, So is *Your praise to the ends of the earth; Your right hand is full of righteousness.*—Psalm 48:10

I will praise You forever, Because You have done it; *And in the presence of Your saints I will wait on Your name, for* it is *good.*—Psalm 52:9

Bless the LORD, O my soul, And forget not all His benefits: Who forgives all your iniquities, Who heals all your diseases,—Psalm 103:2-3

I will sing to the LORD as long as I live; I will sing praise to my God while I have my being. May my meditation be sweet to Him; I will be glad in the LORD.—Psalm 104:33-34

PRIORITIES

Also Jehoshaphat said to the king of Israel, "Please inquire for the word of the LORD today."
—1 Kings 22:5

He who follows righteousness and mercy Finds life, righteousness, and honor.—Proverbs 21:21

Let us hear the conclusion of the whole matter: Fear God and keep His commandments, For this is man's all.—Ecclesiastes 12:13

"No one can serve two masters; for either he will hate the one and love the other, or else he will be loyal to the one and despise the other. You cannot serve God and mammon.—Matthew 6:24

But seek first the kingdom of God and His righteousness, and all these things shall be added to you.—Matthew 6:33

Flee also youthful lusts; but pursue righteousness, faith, love, peace with those who call on the Lord out of a pure heart.—2 Timothy 2:22

PROCEDURES (SEE SURGERY}

PROSPERITY

The keeper of the prison did not look into anything that was *under* Joseph's *authority, because the* LORD *was with him; and whatever he did, the* LORD *made* it *prosper.*—Genesis 39:23

He sought God in the days of Zechariah, who had understanding in the visions of God; and as long as he sought the LORD, *God made him prosper.*
—2 Chronicles 26:5

Blessed is the man Who walks not in the counsel of the ungodly, Nor stands in the path of sinners, Nor sits in the seat of the scornful; But his delight is in the law of the LORD, *And in His law he meditates day and night. He shall be like a tree Planted by the rivers of water, That brings forth its fruit in its season, Whose leaf also shall not wither; And whatever he does shall prosper.*—Psalm 1:1-3

A father of the fatherless, a defender of widows, Is God in His holy habitation. God sets the solitary in families; He brings out those who are bound into prosperity; But the rebellious dwell in a dry land.

—Psalm 68:5-6

Honor the LORD *with your possessions, And with the firstfruits of all your increase; So your barns will be filled with plenty, And your vats will overflow with new wine.*—Proverbs 3:9-10

Bring all the tithes into the storehouse, That there may be food in My house, And try Me now in this," Says the LORD *of hosts, "If I will not open for you the windows of heaven And pour out for you* such *blessing That* there will *not* be room *enough* to receive i*t. "And I will rebuke the devourer for your sakes, So that he will not destroy the fruit of your ground, Nor shall the vine fail to bear fruit for you in the field," Says the* LORD *of hosts;*

—Malachi 3:10-11

Beloved, I pray that you may prosper in all things and be in health, just as your soul prospers.

—3 John 1:2

PROTECTION

The eternal God is your *refuge, And underneath* are *the everlasting arms; He will thrust out the enemy from before you, And will say, 'Destroy!'*
—Deuteronomy 33:27

As for God, His way is perfect; The word of the LORD *is proven; He is a shield to all who trust in Him.*—2 Samuel 22:31

Oh, how great is *Your goodness, Which You have laid up for those who fear You,* Which *You have prepared for those who trust in You In the presence of the sons of men!*—Psalm 31:19

You are *my hiding place; You shall preserve me from trouble; You shall surround me with songs of deliverance.* Selah—Psalm 32:7

For the LORD *loves justice, And does not forsake His saints; They are preserved forever, But the descendants of the wicked shall be cut off.*
—Psalm 37:28

"Because he has set his love upon Me, therefore I will deliver him; I will set him on high, because he has known My name. He shall call upon Me, and I will answer him; I will be *with him in trouble; I will deliver him and honor him.*—Psalm 91:14-15

The LORD preserves all who love Him, But all the wicked He will destroy.—Psalm 145:20

He stores up sound wisdom for the upright; He is a shield to those who walk uprightly; He guards the paths of justice, And preserves the way of His saints.—Proverbs 2:7-8

My Father, who has given them *to Me, is greater than all; and no one is able to snatch* them *out of My Father's hand.*—John 10:29

And the God of peace will crush Satan under your feet shortly. The grace of our Lord Jesus Christ be *with you. Amen.*—Romans 16:20

But the Lord is faithful, who will establish you and guard you *from the evil one.*
—2 Thessalonians 3:3

PURPOSE

The LORD will perfect that which *concerns me; Your mercy, O LORD,* endures *forever; Do not forsake the works of Your hands.*—Psalm 138:8

And we know that all things work together for good to those who love God, to those who are the called according to His *purpose.*—Romans 8:28

For we are His workmanship, created in Christ Jesus for good works, which God prepared beforehand that we should walk in them.—Ephesians 2:10

Therefore we also pray always for you that our God would count you worthy of this *calling, and fulfill all the good pleasure of* His *goodness and the work of faith with power,*—2 Thessalonians 1:11

RECOVERY

I sought the LORD, *and He heard me, And delivered me from all my fears. They looked to Him and were radiant, And their faces were not ashamed. This poor man cried out, and the* LORD *heard* him, *And saved him out of all his troubles. The angel of the* LORD *encamps all around those who fear Him, And delivers them. Oh, taste and see that the* LORD *is good; Blessed* is *the man* who *trusts in Him!*—Psalm 34:4-8

Oh, give thanks to the LORD, *for He is good! For His mercy endures forever. Let the redeemed of the* LORD *say so, Whom He has redeemed from the hand of the enemy. Then they cried out to the* LORD *in their trouble, And He delivered them out of their distresses.*—Psalm 107:1-2,6

REDEMPTION

You drew near on the day I called on You, And said, "Do not fear!" O Lord, You have pleaded the case for my soul; You have redeemed my life.
                    —Lamentations 3:57-58

I have blotted out, like a thick cloud, your transgressions, And like a cloud, your sins. Return to Me, for I have redeemed you."—Isaiah 44:22

But of Him you are in Christ Jesus, who became for us wisdom from God—and righteousness and sanctification and redemption— —1 Corinthians 1:30

In Him we have redemption through His blood, the forgiveness of sins, according to the riches of His grace—Ephesians 1:7

He has delivered us from the power of darkness and conveyed us into the kingdom of the Son of His love, in whom we have redemption through His blood, the forgiveness of sins.—Colossians 1:13-14

knowing that you were not redeemed with corruptible things, like *silver or gold, from your aimless conduct* received *by tradition from your fathers, but with the precious blood of Christ, as of a lamb without blemish and without spot.*—1 Peter 1:18-19

REFUGE

Be merciful to me, O God, be merciful to me! For my soul trusts in You; And in the shadow of Your wings I will make my refuge, Until these *calamities have passed by. I will cry out to God Most High, To God who performs* all things *for me.*

—Psalm 57:1-2

REPENTANCE

Let the wicked forsake his way, And the unrighteous man his thoughts; Let him return to the LORD, *And He will have mercy on him; And to our God, For He will abundantly pardon.*—Isaiah 55:7

"But if a wicked man turns from all his sins which he has committed, keeps all My statutes, and does what is lawful and right, he shall surely live; he shall not die.—Ezekiel 18:21

I say to you that likewise there will be more joy in heaven over one sinner who repents than over ninety-nine just persons who need no repentance.

—Luke 15:7

Repent therefore and be converted, that your sins may be blotted out, so that times of refreshing may come from the presence of the Lord,—Acts 3:19

The Lord is not slack concerning His *promise, as some count slackness, but is longsuffering toward us, not willing that any should perish but that all should come to repentance.*—2 Peter 3:9

REST

The LORD *will fight for you, and you shall hold your peace."*—Exodus 14:14

"Teach me, and I will hold my tongue; Cause me to understand wherein I have erred.—Job 6:24

I will both lie down in peace, and sleep; For You alone, O LORD, *make me dwell in safety.*
—Psalm 4:8

According to Your name, O God, So is Your praise to the ends of the earth; Your right hand is full of righteousness.—Psalm 48:10

Truly my soul silently waits for God; From Him comes my salvation. He only is my rock and my salvation; He is my defense; I shall not be greatly moved.—Psalm 62:1-2

The fear of the LORD *leads to life, And* he who has it *will abide in satisfaction; He will not be visited with evil.*—Proverbs 19:23

Come to Me, all you *who labor and are heavy laden, and I will give you rest. Take My yoke upon you and learn from Me, for I am gentle and lowly in heart, and you will find rest for your souls. For My yoke* is *easy and My burden is light."*

—Matthew 11:28-30

For we who have believed do enter that rest, as He has said: "So I swore in My wrath, 'They shall not enter My rest,'" although the works were finished from the foundation of the world.—Hebrews 4:3

RESURRECTION POWER

Heal the sick, cleanse the lepers, raise the dead, cast out demons. Freely you have received, freely give.

—Matthew 10:8

When He came in, He said to them, "Why make this commotion and weep? The child is not dead, but sleeping." Then He took the child by the hand, and said to her, "Talitha, cumi," which is translated, "Little girl, I say to you, arise."—Mark 5:39,41

*Jesus said to her, "Your brother will rise again."
Then they took away the stone from the place where
the dead man was lying. And Jesus lifted up His
eyes and said, "Father, I thank You that You have
heard Me. And I know that You always hear Me,
but because of the people who are standing by I said
this, that they may believe that You sent Me." Now
when He had said these things, He cried with a loud
voice, "Lazarus, come forth!" And he who had died
came out bound hand and foot with grave clothes,
and his face was wrapped with a cloth. Jesus said to
them, "Loose him, and let him go."*
—John 11:23,41-44

REVEAL SECRETS

*'Call to Me, and I will answer you, and show you
great and mighty things, which you do not know.'*
—Jeremiah 33:3

REVIVE

*Come, and let us return to the LORD; for He has
torn, but He will heal us; He has stricken, but He
will bind us up. After two days He will revive us; on
the third day He will raise us up, that we may live
in His sight.*—Hosea 6:1-2

REWARD

The LORD rewarded me according to my righteousness; According to the cleanness of my hands He has recompensed me.—Psalm 18:20

I, the LORD, search the heart, I test the mind, Even to give every man according to his ways, According to the fruit of his doings.—Jeremiah 17:10

But you, when you pray, go into your room, and when you have shut your door, pray to your Father who is in the secret place; and your Father who sees in secret will reward you openly.—Matthew 6:6

But love your enemies, do good, and lend, hoping for nothing in return; and your reward will be great, and you will be sons of the Most High. For He is kind to the unthankful and evil.—Luke 6:35

And whatever you do, do it heartily, as to the Lord and not to men, knowing that from the Lord you will receive the reward of the inheritance; for you serve the Lord Christ.—Colossians 3:23-24

"And behold, I am coming quickly, and My reward is with Me, to give to every one according to his work.—Revelation 22:12

RIGHTEOUSNESS

Surely he will never be shaken; The righteous will be in everlasting remembrance. He will not be afraid of evil tidings; His heart is steadfast, trusting in the LORD.—Psalm 112:6-7

In the way of righteousness is life, And in its pathway there is no death.—Proverbs 12:28

The work of righteousness will be peace, And the effect of righteousness, quietness and assurance forever.—Isaiah 32:17

Sow for yourselves righteousness; Reap in mercy; Break up your fallow ground, For it is time to seek the LORD, *Till He comes and rains righteousness on you.*—Hosea 10:12

For the eyes of the LORD *are on the righteous, And His ears are open to their prayers; But the face of the* LORD *is against those who do evil."*
　　　　　　　　　　—1 Peter 3:12

SAFETY

"Because he has set his love upon Me, therefore I will deliver him; I will set him on high, because he has known My name. He shall call upon Me, and I will answer him; I will be *with him in trouble; I will deliver him and honor him.*—Psalm 91:14-15

The LORD *will perfect* that which *concerns me; Your mercy, O* LORD, endures *forever; Do not forsake the works of Your hands.*—Psalm 138:8

The name of the LORD is *a strong tower; The righteous run to it and are safe.*—Proverbs 18:10

But thus says the LORD: *"Even the captives of the mighty shall be taken away, And the prey of the terrible be delivered; For I will contend with him who contends with you, And I will save your children.*
—Isaiah 49:25

SALVATION

Truly my soul silently waits for God; From Him comes my salvation. He only is my rock and my salvation; He is my defense; I shall not be greatly moved.—Psalm 62:1-2

In God is *my salvation and my glory; The rock of my strength,* And *my refuge,* is *in God.*
—Psalm 62:7

And she will bring forth a Son, and you shall call His name JESUS, for He will save His people from their sins."—Matthew 1:21

For I am not ashamed of the gospel of Christ, for it is the power of God to salvation for everyone who believes, for the Jew first and also for the Greek.
—Romans 1:16

that if you confess with your mouth the Lord Jesus and believe in your heart that God has raised Him from the dead, you will be saved.—Romans 10:9

For He made Him who knew no sin to be sin for us, that we might become the righteousness of God in Him.—2 Corinthians 5:21

For He says: "In an acceptable time I have heard you, And in the day of salvation I have helped you." Behold, now is *the accepted time; behold, now* is *the day of salvation.*—2 Corinthians 6:2

I have been crucified with Christ; it is no longer I who live, but Christ lives in me; and the life *which I now live in the flesh I live by faith in the Son of God, who loved me and gave Himself for me.*
—Galatians 2:20

But when the fullness of the time had come, God sent forth His Son, born of a woman, born under the law, to redeem those who were under the law, that we might receive the adoption as sons. And because you are sons, God has sent forth the Spirit of His Son into your hearts, crying out, "Abba, Father!" Therefore you are no longer a slave but a son, and if a son, then an heir of God through Christ.

—Galatians 4:4-7

But let us who are of the day be sober, putting on the breastplate of faith and love, and as *a helmet the hope of salvation*—1 Thessalonians 5:8

For the grace of God that brings salvation has appeared to all men, teaching us that, denying ungodliness and worldly lusts, we should live soberly, righteously, and godly in the present age,

—Titus 2:11-12

And having been perfected, He became the author of eternal salvation to all who obey Him,

—Hebrews 5:9

Save

Now I know that the LORD saves His anointed; He will answer him from His holy heaven With the saving strength of His right hand. Some trust *in chariots, and some in horses; But we will remember the name of the LORD our God. They have bowed down and fallen; But we have risen and stand upright. Save, LORD! May the King answer us when we call.*—Psalm 20:6-9

The LORD is near to all who call upon Him, To all who call upon Him in truth. He will fulfill the desire of those who fear Him; He also will hear their cry and save them.—Psalm 145:18-19

He who believes and is baptized will be saved; but he who does not believe will be condemned.

—Mark 16:16

The thief does not come except to steal, and to kill, and to destroy. I have come that they may have life, and that they may have it *more abundantly.*

—John 10:10

And if anyone hears My words and does not believe, I do not judge him; for I did not come to judge the world but to save the world.—John 12:47

So they said, "Believe on the Lord Jesus Christ, and you will be saved, you and your household."
—Acts 16:31

that if you confess with your mouth the Lord Jesus and believe in your heart that God has raised Him from the dead, you will be saved.—Romans 10:9

For this is *good and acceptable in the sight of God our Savior, who desires all men to be saved and to come to the knowledge of the truth.*
—1 Timothy 2:3-4

who has saved us and called us with a holy calling, not according to our works, but according to His own purpose and grace which was given to us in Christ Jesus before time began,—2 Timothy 1:9

not by works of righteousness which we have done, but according to His mercy He saved us, through the washing of regeneration and renewing of the Holy Spirit, whom He poured out on us abundantly through Jesus Christ our Savior, that having been justified by His grace we should become heirs according to the hope of eternal life.—Titus 3:5-7

Therefore lay aside all filthiness and overflow of wickedness, and receive with meekness the implanted word, which is able to save your souls.
—James 1:21

And this is the testimony: that God has given us eternal life, and this life is in His Son. He who has the Son has life; he who does not have the Son of God does not have life.—1 John 5:11-12

SCRIPTURES

This Book of the Law shall not depart from your mouth, but you shall meditate in it day and night, that you may observe to do according to all that is written in it. For then you will make your way prosperous, and then you will have good success.
—Joshua 1:8

For whatever things were written before were written for our learning, that we through the patience and comfort of the Scriptures might have hope.
—Romans 15:4

All Scripture is given by inspiration of God, and is profitable for doctrine, for reproof, for correction, for instruction in righteousness, that the man of God may be complete, thoroughly equipped for every good work.—2 Timothy 3:16-17

For the word of God is living and powerful, and sharper than any two-edged sword, piercing even to the division of soul and spirit, and of joints and marrow, and is a discerner of the thoughts and intents of the heart.—Hebrews 4:12

SECURITY

Of Benjamin he said: "The beloved of the LORD shall dwell in safety by Him, Who shelters him all the day long; And he shall dwell between His shoulders."—Deuteronomy 33:12

O LORD, You are the portion of my inheritance and my cup; You maintain my lot.—Psalm 16:5

Behold, I will bring it health and healing; I will heal them and reveal to them the abundance of peace and truth.—Jeremiah 33:6

And I give them eternal life, and they shall never perish; neither shall anyone snatch them out of My hand.—John 10:28

So we may boldly say: The LORD is my helper; I will not fear. What can man do to me?"
—Hebrews 13:6

SEIZURES

News about him spread all over Syria, and people brought to him all who were ill with various diseases, those suffering severe pain, the demon-possessed, those having seizures, and the paralyzed, and he healed them.—Matthew 4:24 NIV

SELF-CONTROL

No temptation has overtaken you except such as is common to man; but God is faithful, who will not allow you to be tempted beyond what you are able, but with the temptation will also make the way of escape, that you may be able to bear it.

—1 Corinthians 10:13

For the grace of God that brings salvation has appeared to all men, teaching us that, denying ungodliness and worldly lusts, we should live soberly, righteously, and godly in the present age,

—Titus 2:11-12

Therefore gird up the loins of your mind, be sober, and rest your hope fully upon the grace that is to be brought to you at the revelation of Jesus Christ;

—1 Peter 1:13

But the end of all things is at hand; therefore be serious and watchful in your prayers.—1 Peter 4:7

Be sober, be vigilant; because your adversary the devil walks about like a roaring lion, seeking whom he may devour.—1 Peter 5:8

SICKNESS

So you shall serve the LORD your God, and He will bless your bread and your water. And I will take sickness away from the midst of you.
—Exodus 23:25

Therefore you shall keep the commandment, the statutes, and the judgments which I command you today, to observe them. Then it shall come to pass, because you listen to these judgments, and keep and do them, that the LORD your God will keep with you the covenant and the mercy which He swore to your fathers. And the LORD will take away from you all sickness, and will afflict you with none of the terrible diseases of Egypt which you have known, but will lay them *on all those who hate you.*
—Deuteronomy 7:11-12,15

The LORD will strengthen him on his bed of illness; You will sustain him on his sickbed.—Psalm 41:3

And Jesus went about all Galilee, teaching in their synagogues, preaching the gospel of the kingdom, and healing all kinds of sickness and all kinds of disease among the people. Then His fame went throughout all Syria; and they brought to Him all sick people who were afflicted with various diseases and torments, and those who were demon-possessed, epileptics, and paralytics; and He healed them.
—Matthew 4:23-24

Then Jesus went about all the cities and villages, teaching in their synagogues, preaching the gospel of the kingdom, and healing every sickness and every disease among the people.—Matthew 9:35

And when He had called His twelve disciples to Him, *He gave them power* over *unclean spirits, to cast them out, and to heal all kinds of sickness and all kinds of disease.*—Matthew 10:1

And when Jesus went out He saw a great multitude; and He was moved with compassion for them, and healed their sick.—Matthew 14:14

Then He healed many who were sick with various diseases, and cast out many demons; and He did not allow the demons to speak, because they knew Him.—Mark 1:34

and to have power to heal sicknesses and to cast out demons:—Mark 3:15

And they cast out many demons, and anointed with oil many who were sick, and healed them.
—Mark 6:13

When the sun was setting, all those who had any that were sick with various diseases brought them to Him; and He laid His hands on every one of them and healed them.—Luke 4:40

However, the report went around concerning Him all the more; and great multitudes came together to hear, and to be healed by Him of their infirmities.
—Luke 5:15

So when he heard about Jesus, he sent elders of the Jews to Him, pleading with Him to come and heal his servant. Therefore I did not even think myself worthy to come to You. But say the word, and my servant will be healed. And those who were sent, returning to the house, found the servant well who had been sick.—Luke 7:3,7,10

He sent them to preach the kingdom of God and to heal the sick.—Luke 9:2

And heal the sick there, and say to them, 'The kingdom of God has come near to you.'
—Luke 10:9

Also a multitude gathered from the surrounding cities to Jerusalem, bringing sick people and those who were tormented by unclean spirits, and they were all healed.—Acts 5:16

Is anyone among you suffering? Let him pray. Is anyone cheerful? Let him sing psalms. Is anyone among you sick? Let him call for the elders of the church, and let them pray over him, anointing him with oil in the name of the Lord. And the prayer of faith will save the sick, and the Lord will raise him up. And if he has committed sins, he will be forgiven. Confess your trespasses to one another, and pray for one another, that you may be healed. The effective, fervent prayer of a righteous man avails much.—James 5:13-16

SIGHT

Moses was one hundred and twenty years old when he died. His eyes were not dim nor his natural vigor diminished.—Deuteronomy 34:7

They said to Him, "Lord, that our eyes may be opened." So Jesus had compassion and touched their eyes. And immediately their eyes received sight, and they followed Him.—Matthew 20:33-34

Then He put His hands on his eyes again and made him look up. And he was restored and saw everyone clearly.—Mark 8:25

And Jesus said, "For judgment I have come into this world, that those who do not see may see ...
—John 9:39

Jesus said to her, "Did I not say to you that if you would believe you would see the glory of God?"
—John 11:40

SKIN

So he went down and dipped seven times in the Jordan, according to the saying of the man of God; and his flesh was restored like the flesh of a little child, and he was clean.—2 Kings 5:14

SLEEP

And you will have confidence, because there is hope; you will be protected and take your rest in safety. You will lie down, and none will make you afraid; many will entreat your favor.
—Job 11:18-19 RSV

When you lie down, you will not be afraid; Yes, you will lie down and your sleep will be sweet.
—Proverbs 3:24

SNAKE BITE

they will take up serpents; and if they drink any-thing deadly, it will by no means hurt them; they will lay hands on the sick, and they will recover."
                                    —Mark 16:18

SORROW

And Jehovah said, I have surely seen the affliction of my people ... and have heard their cry ... for I know their sorrows; and I am come down to deliver them ...—Exodus 3:7-8 ASV

But I am poor and sorrowful; Let Your salvation, O God, set me up on high.—Psalm 69:29

I love the LORD, because He has heard My voice and my supplications. Because He has inclined His ear to me, Therefore I will call upon Him as long as I live. The pains of death surrounded me, And the pangs of Sheol laid hold of me; I found trouble and sorrow. Then I called upon the name of the LORD: "O LORD, I implore You, deliver my soul!" Gracious is the LORD, and righteous; Yes, our God is merciful. The LORD preserves the simple; I was brought low, and He saved me. Return to your rest, O my soul, For the LORD has dealt bountifully with you. For You have delivered my soul from death, My eyes from tears, And my feet from falling. I will walk before the LORD In the land of the living.—Psalm 116:1-9

It shall come to pass in the day the LORD gives you rest from your sorrow, and from your fear and the hard bondage in which you were made to serve.
          —Isaiah 14:3

So the ransomed of the LORD shall return, and come to Zion with singing, with everlasting joy on their heads. They shall obtain joy and gladness; sorrow and sighing shall flee away.—Isaiah 51:11

Surely He has borne our griefs and carried our sorrows; yet we esteemed Him stricken, smitten by God, and afflicted.—Isaiah 53:4

SPEAKING

Now therefore, go, and I will be with your mouth and teach you what you shall say" Now you shall speak to him and put the words in his mouth. And I will be with your mouth and with his mouth, and I will teach you what you shall do.
          —Exodus 4:12,15

The LORD will fight for you, and you shall hold your peace."—Exodus 14:14

"Teach me, and I will hold my tongue; Cause me to understand wherein I have erred.—Job 6:24

Death and life are *in the power of the tongue, And those who love it will eat its fruit.*
—Proverbs 18:21

And I have put My words in your mouth; I have covered you with the shadow of My hand …
—Isaiah 51:16

STABILITY

I have set the LORD always before me; Because He is *at my right hand I shall not be moved.*
—Psalm 16:8

For they shall soon be cut down like the grass, And wither as the green herb. Trust in the LORD, and do good; Dwell in the land, and feed on His faithfulness.—Psalm 37:2-3

He who walks with integrity walks securely, But he who perverts his ways will become known.
—Proverbs 10:9

Strengthen the weak hands, And make firm the feeble knees. Say to those who are *fearful-hearted, "Be strong, do not fear! Behold, your God will come* with *vengeance,* With *the recompense of God; He will come and save you."*—Isaiah 35:3-4

Fear not, for I am with you; Be not dismayed, for I am your God. I will strengthen you, Yes, I will help you, I will uphold you with My righteous right hand.'—Isaiah 41:10

But may the God of all grace, who called us to His eternal glory by Christ Jesus, after you have suffered a while, perfect, establish, strengthen, and settle you.—1 Peter 5:10

He who loves his brother abides in the light, and there is no cause for stumbling in him.
—1 John 2:10

Now to Him who is able to keep you from stumbling, And to present you *faultless Before the presence of His glory with exceeding joy, To God our Savior, Who alone is wise,* Be *glory and majesty, Dominion and power, Both now and forever. Amen.*—Jude 1:24-25

STAND

He also brought me up out of a horrible pit, Out of the miry clay, And set my feet upon a rock, And established my steps.—Psalm 40:2

And He said to me, "Son of man, stand on your feet, and I will speak to you."—Ezekiel 2:1

And behold, there was a woman who had a spirit of infirmity eighteen years, and was bent over and could in no way raise herself up. But when Jesus saw her, He called her to Him and said to her, "Woman, you are loosed from your infirmity." And He laid His hands on her, and immediately she was made straight, and glorified God.—Luke 13:11-13

STRENGTH

The LORD is my strength and song, And He has become my salvation; He is my God, and I will praise Him; My father's God, and I will exalt Him.—Exodus 15:2

God is my strength and power, And He makes my way perfect. He makes my feet like the feet of deer, And sets me on my high places.
—2 Samuel 22:33-34

Now I know that the LORD saves His anointed; He will answer him from His holy heaven With the saving strength of His right hand. Some trust in chariots, and some in horses; But we will remember the name of the LORD our God. They have bowed down and fallen; But we have risen and stand upright. Save, LORD! May the King answer us when we call.—Psalm 20:6-9

The LORD is my light and my salvation; Whom shall I fear? The LORD is the strength of my life; Of whom shall I be afraid?—Psalm 27:1

Jehovah will give strength unto his people; Jehovah will bless his people with peace.
—Psalm 29:11 ASV

Be of good courage, And He shall strengthen your heart, All you who hope in the LORD.
—Psalm 31:24

My flesh and my heart fail; But God is the strength of my heart and my portion forever.—Psalm 73:26

He gives power to the weak, And to those who have no might He increases strength.
—Isaiah 40:29

Fear not, for I am with you; Be not dismayed, for I am your God. I will strengthen you, Yes, I will help you, I will uphold you with My righteous right hand.'—Isaiah 41:10

"I will seek what was lost and bring back what was driven away, bind up the broken and strengthen what was sick; but I will destroy the fat and the strong, and feed them in judgment."
—Ezekiel 34:16

Beat your plowshares into swords And your pruning hooks into spears; Let the weak say, 'I am strong.'"—Joel 3:10

And He said to me, "My grace is sufficient for you, for My strength is made perfect in weakness." Therefore most gladly I will rather boast in my infirmities, that the power of Christ may rest upon me.
                    —2 Corinthians 12:9

Finally, my brethren, be strong in the Lord and in the power of His might.—Ephesians 6:10

I can do all things through Christ who strengthens me.—Philippians 4:13

SUFFERING

Remember your word to your servant, for you have given me hope. My comfort in my suffering is this: Your promise preserves my life.
                    —Psalm 119:49-50 NIV

He said to her, "Daughter, your faith has healed you. Go in peace and be freed from your suffering."—Mark 5:34 NIV

who, in the days of His flesh, when He had offered up prayers and supplications, with vehement cries and tears to Him who was able to save Him from death, and was heard because of His godly fear, though He was a Son, yet He learned obedience by the things which He suffered.—Hebrews 5:7-8

SURGERY (BEFORE ANY PROCEDURES)

In God I have put my trust; I will not be afraid. What can man do to me?—Psalm 56:11

He who dwells in the secret place of the Most High Shall abide under the shadow of the Almighty. I will say of the LORD, "He is my refuge and my fortress; My God, in Him I will trust." Surely He shall deliver you from the snare of the fowler And *from the perilous pestilence. He shall cover you with His feathers, And under His wings you shall take refuge; His truth* shall be your *shield and buckler. You shall not be afraid of the terror by night,* Nor *of the arrow* that *flies by day,* Nor *of the pestilence* that *walks in darkness,* Nor *of the destruction* that *lays waste at noonday. A thousand may fall at your side, And ten thousand at your right hand;* But *it shall not come near you. Only with your eyes shall you look, And see the reward of the wicked. Because you have made the LORD,* who is *my refuge,* Even *the Most High, your dwelling place, No evil shall befall you, Nor shall any plague come near your dwelling; For He shall give His angels charge over you, To keep you in all your ways. In their hands they shall bear you up, Lest you dash your foot against a stone. You shall tread upon the lion and the cobra, The young lion and the serpent you shall trample under-*

foot. "Because he has set his love upon Me, therefore I will deliver him; I will set him on high, because he has known My name. He shall call upon Me, and I will answer him; I will be *with him in trouble; I will deliver him and honor him. With long life I will satisfy him, And show him My salvation."*

—Psalm 91

Bless the LORD, *O my soul; And all that is within me,* bless *His holy name! Bless the* LORD, *O my soul, And forget not all His benefits: Who forgives all your iniquities, Who heals all your diseases, Who redeems your life from destruction, Who crowns you with lovingkindness and tender mercies, Who satisfies your mouth with good* things, *So* that *your youth is renewed like the eagle's.*—Psalm 103:1-5

But now, thus says the LORD, *who created you, O Jacob, And He who formed you, O Israel: "Fear not, for I have redeemed you; I have called you by your name; You are Mine. When you pass through the waters, I will be with you; And through the rivers, they shall not overflow you. When you walk through the fire, you shall not be burned, Nor shall the flame scorch you. For I am the* LORD *your God, The Holy One of Israel, your Savior; I gave Egypt for your ransom, Ethiopia and Seba in your place.*—Isaiah 43:1-3

Then your light shall break forth like the morning, Your healing shall spring forth speedily, And your righteousness shall go before you; The glory of the LORD shall be your rear guard. Then you shall call, and the LORD will answer; You shall cry, and He will say, 'Here I am.' "If you take away the yoke from your midst, The pointing of the finger, and speaking wickedness,—Isaiah 58:8-9

THIRSTY

On the last day, that great day *of the feast, Jesus stood and cried out, saying, "If anyone thirsts, let him come to Me and drink. He who believes in Me, as the Scripture has said, out of his heart will flow rivers of living water."*—John 7:37-38

THANKFULNESS

Oh, give thanks to the LORD! Call upon His name; Make known His deeds among the peoples! Sing to Him, sing psalms to Him; Talk of all His wondrous works!—1 Chronicles 16:8-9

Oh, give thanks to the LORD, for He *is good! For His mercy* endures *forever.*—Chronicles 16:34

The LORD is my strength and my shield; My heart trusted in Him, and I am helped; Therefore my heart greatly rejoices, And with my song I will praise Him.—Psalm 28:7

You have turned for me my mourning into dancing; You have put off my sackcloth and clothed me with gladness, To the end that my *glory may sing praise to You and not be silent. O LORD my God, I will give thanks to You forever.*—Psalm 30:11-12

Oh, that men *would give thanks to the LORD for His goodness, And* for *His wonderful works to the children of men! For He satisfies the longing soul, And fills the hungry soul with goodness.*
—Psalm 107:8-9

I know that the LORD will maintain The cause of the afflicted, And *justice for the poor. Surely the righteous shall give thanks to Your name; The upright shall dwell in Your presence.*
—Psalm 140:12-13

And Jesus took the loaves, and when He had given thanks He distributed them *to the disciples, and the disciples to those sitting down; and likewise of the fish, as much as they wanted.*—John 6:11

As you therefore have received Christ Jesus the Lord, so walk in Him, rooted and built up in Him and established in the faith, as you have been taught, abounding in it with thanksgiving.

—Colossians 2:6-7

in everything give thanks; for this is the will of God in Christ Jesus for you.—1 Thessalonians 5:18

THOUGHTS

Search me, O God, and know my heart; Try me, and know my anxieties; And see if there is any wicked way in me, And lead me in the way everlasting.—Psalm 139:23-24

Every way of a man is *right in his own eyes, But the* LORD *weighs the hearts.*—Proverbs 21:2

Let the wicked forsake his way, And the unrighteous man his thoughts; Let him return to the LORD, *And He will have mercy on him; And to our God, For He will abundantly pardon. "For My thoughts* are *not your thoughts, Nor* are *your ways My ways," says the* LORD.—Isaiah 55:7-8

And do not be conformed to this world, but be transformed by the renewing of your mind, that you may prove what is *that good and acceptable and perfect will of God.*—Romans 12:2

For "who has known the mind of the LORD that he may instruct Him?" But we have the mind of Christ.—1 Corinthians 2:16

Let no one deceive himself. If anyone among you seems to be wise in this age, let him become a fool that he may become wise.—1 Corinthians 3:18

casting down arguments and every high thing that exalts itself against the knowledge of God, bringing every thought into captivity to the obedience of Christ,—2 Corinthians 10:5

and be renewed in the spirit of your mind,
—Ephesians 4:23

Finally, brethren, whatever things are true, whatever things are noble, whatever things are just, whatever things are pure, whatever things are lovely, whatever things are of good report, if there is any virtue and if there is anything praiseworthy—meditate on these things.—Philippians 4:8

For the word of God is living and powerful, and sharper than any two-edged sword, piercing even to the division of soul and spirit, and of joints and marrow, and is a discerner of the thoughts and intents of the heart.—Hebrews 4:12

TIRED

Have you not known? Have you not heard? The everlasting God, the LORD, The Creator of the ends of the earth, Neither faints nor is weary. His understanding is unsearchable. He gives power to the weak And to those who have *no might He increases strength.*—Isaiah 40:28-29

Even the youths shall faint and be weary, And the young men shall utterly fall, But those who wait on the LORD Shall renew their *strength; They shall mount up with wings like eagles, They shall run and not be weary, They shall walk and not faint.*
—Isaiah 40:30-31

TRIAL

Blessed is the man who endures temptation; for when he has been approved, he will receive the crown of life which the Lord has promised to those who love Him.—James 1:12

TRUST

And those who know Your name will put their trust in You; For You, LORD, have not forsaken those who seek You.—Psalm 9:10

Oh, taste and see that the LORD is good; Blessed is the man who trusts in Him!—Psalm 34:8

Commit your way to the LORD, Trust also in Him, And He shall bring it to pass.—Psalm 37:5

Blessed is that man who makes the LORD his trust, And does not respect the proud, nor such as turn aside to lies.—Psalm 40:4

Whenever I am afraid, I will trust in You. In God (I will praise His word), In God I have put my trust; I will not fear. What can flesh do to me?
—Psalm 56:3-4

It is better to trust in the LORD Than to put confidence in man. It is better to trust in the LORD Than to put confidence in princes.
—Psalm 118:8-9

Those who trust in the LORD Are like Mount Zion, Which cannot be moved, but abides forever.
—Psalm 125:1

And *so find favor and high esteem In the sight of God and man. Trust in the* LORD *with all your heart, And lean not on your own understanding; In all your ways acknowledge Him, And He shall direct your paths. Do not be wise in your own eyes; Fear the* LORD *and depart from evil. It will be health to your flesh, And strength to your bones.*
—Proverbs 3:4-8

You will keep him *in perfect peace,* Whose *mind* is *stayed* on You, *Because he trusts in You. Trust in the* LORD *forever, For in* YAH, *the* LORD, is *everlasting strength.*—Isaiah 26:3-4

For thus says the LORD GOD, *the Holy One of Israel: "In returning and rest you shall be saved; In quietness and confidence shall be your strength." But you would not,*—Isaiah 30:15

"Who among you fears the LORD? *Who obeys the voice of His Servant? Who walks in darkness And has no light? Let him trust in the name of the* LORD *And rely upon his God.*—Isaiah 50:10

"Blessed is *the man who trusts in the* LORD, *And whose hope is the* LORD. *For he shall be like a tree planted by the waters, Which spreads out its roots by the river, And will not fear when heat comes; But its leaf will be green, And will not be anxious in the year of drought, Nor will cease from yielding fruit.*
—Jeremiah 17:7-8

The LORD is good, A stronghold in the day of trouble; And He knows those who trust in Him.
—Nahum 1:7

"Let not your heart be troubled; you believe in God, believe also in Me.—John 14:1

WALK

Then behold, they brought to Him a paralytic lying on a bed. When Jesus saw their faith, He said to the paralytic, "Son, be of good cheer; your sins are forgiven you." And at once some of the scribes said within themselves, "This Man blasphemes!" But Jesus, knowing their thoughts, said, "Why do you think evil in your hearts? For which is easier, to say, 'Your sins are forgiven you,' or to say, 'Arise and walk'? But that you may know that the Son of Man has power on earth to forgive sins"—then He said to the paralytic, "Arise, take up your bed, and go to your house." And he arose and departed to his house.—Matthew 9:2-7

Jesus said to him, "Rise, take up your bed and walk." And immediately the man was made well, took up his bed, and walked. And that day was the Sabbath.—John 5:8-9

Then Peter said, "Silver and gold I do not have, but what I do have I give you: In the name of Jesus Christ of Nazareth, rise up and walk." And he took him by the right hand and lifted him *up, and immediately his feet and ankle bones received strength. So he, leaping up, stood and walked and entered the temple with them—walking, leaping, and praising God.*—Acts 3:6-8

WISDOM

I will instruct you and teach you in the way you should go; I will guide you with My eye. Do not be like the horse or like the mule, Which have no understanding, Which must be harnessed with bit and bridle, Else they will not come near you.
—Psalm 32:8-9

So teach us *to number our days, That we may gain a heart of wisdom.*—Psalm 90:12

The fear of the LORD *is the beginning of wisdom; A good understanding have all those who do His commandments. His praise endures forever.*
Psalm 111:10

Wisdom is the principal thing; Therefore get wisdom. And in all your getting, get understanding.
—Proverbs 4:7

Give instruction *to a wise* man, *and he will be still wiser; Teach a just* man, *and he will increase in learning.*—Proverbs 9:9

How much better to get wisdom than gold! And to get understanding is to be chosen rather than silver.
                                    —Proverbs 16:16

So shall *the knowledge of wisdom* be *to your soul; If you have found* it, *there is a prospect, And your hope will not be cut off.*—Proverbs 24:14

Wisdom is good with an inheritance, And profitable to those who see the sun. For wisdom is a defense as money is a defense, But the excellence of knowledge is that wisdom gives life to those who have it.
                                    —Ecclesiastes 7:11-12

But the Helper, the Holy Spirit, whom the Father will send in My name, He will teach you all things, and bring to your remembrance all things that I said to you.—John 14:26

For this reason we also, since the day we heard it, do not cease to pray for you, and to ask that you may be filled with the knowledge of His will in all wisdom and spiritual understanding;—Colossians 1:9

Let the word of Christ dwell in you richly in all wisdom, teaching and admonishing one another in psalms and hymns and spiritual songs, singing with grace in your hearts to the Lord.

—Colossians 3:16

If any of you lacks wisdom, let him ask of God, who gives to all liberally and without reproach, and it will be given to him.—James 1:5

But the wisdom that is from above is first pure, then peaceable, gentle, willing to yield, full of mercy and good fruits, without partiality and without hypocrisy.—James 3:17

WORRY

Therefore do not worry about tomorrow, for tomorrow will worry about its own things. Sufficient for the day is *its own trouble.*—Matthew 6:34

For I am persuaded that neither death nor life, nor angels nor principalities nor powers, nor things present nor things to come, nor height nor depth, nor any other created thing, shall be able to separate us from the love of God which is in Christ Jesus our Lord.—Romans 8:38-39

WOUNDS

He heals the brokenhearted And binds up their wounds.—Psalm 147:3

… In the day that the LORD binds up the bruise of His people And heals the stroke of their wound.
—Isaiah 30:26

For I will restore health to you And heal you of your wounds,' says the LORD, …—Jeremiah 30:17

But Jesus answered and said, "Permit even this." And He touched his ear and healed him.
—Luke 22:51

Mark 16:15-18 tells us Jesus commissioned His disciples to preach the Gospel, heal the sick and cast out demons.

John 14:17-20 tells us He told them that they would do greater works than His.

Luke 4:18 tells us the Lord has given us the same commission—to lay hands on the sick, release the captives and set the oppressed free.

Hebrews 13:8 tells us Jesus is still the healer! Jesus Christ the same yesterday and today and forever.

We too are commissioned and empowered as we come to Him.

AUTHORITY OVER SATAN

And when He had called His twelve disciples to Him, He gave them power over unclean spirits, to cast them out, and to heal all kinds of sickness and all kinds of disease.—Matthew 10:1

And He said to them, "I saw Satan fall like lightning from heaven. Behold, I give you the authority to trample on serpents and scorpions, and over all the power of the enemy, and nothing shall by any means hurt you.
—Luke 10:18-19

Now is the judgment of this world; now the ruler of this world will be cast out.—John 12:31

how God anointed Jesus of Nazareth with the Holy Spirit and with power, who went about doing good and healing all who were oppressed by the devil, for God was with Him.—Acts 10:38

I will deliver you from the Jewish *people, as well as* from *the Gentiles, to whom I now send you, to open their eyes,* in order *to turn* them *from darkness to light, and* from *the power of Satan to God, that they may receive forgiveness of sins and an inheritance among those who are sanctified by faith in Me.'*
—Acts 26:17-18

COMMANDED AND EMPOWERED TO HEAL

And when He had called His twelve disciples to Him, *He gave them power* over *unclean spirits, to cast them out, and to heal all kinds of sickness and all kinds of disease. And as you go, preach, saying, 'The kingdom of heaven is at hand.' Heal the sick, cleanse the lepers, raise the dead, cast out demons. Freely you have received, freely give.*—Matthew 10:1,7-8

Then He called His twelve disciples together and gave them power and authority over all demons, and to cure diseases. He sent them to preach the kingdom of God and to heal the sick. So they departed and went through the towns, preaching the gospel and healing everywhere.
—Luke 9:1-2,6

After these things the Lord appointed seventy others also, and sent them two by two before His face into every city and place where He Himself was about to go. And heal the sick there, and say to them, 'The kingdom of God has come near to you.'—Luke 10:1,9

Then Peter said, "Silver and gold I do not have, but what I do have I give you: In the name of Jesus Christ of Nazareth, rise up and walk." And he took him by the right hand and lifted him *up, and immediately his feet and ankle bones received strength. So he, leaping up, stood and walked and entered the temple with them— walking, leaping, and praising God.*—Acts 3:6-8

COMFORT DURING SUFFERING

This is *my comfort in my affliction, For Your word has given me life.*—Psalm 119:50

Surely He has borne our griefs And carried our sorrows; yet we esteemed Him stricken, Smitten by God, and afflicted. But He was *wounded for our transgressions,* He was *bruised for our iniquities; The chastisement for our peace* was *upon Him, And by His stripes we are healed.*—Isaiah 53:4-5

PRAYER FOR THE SICK

Dear Father,

Today we come boldly before Your throne of grace at Your invitation. You have promised that where two or more are gathered, there You will be in the midst of them. So we come today in agreement, confessing Your Word concerning healing for _____ in the name of Jesus, asking for Your presence and blessing. We know that because of Jesus' suffering there was victory at the cross for us. As we come to You asking forgiveness of our sins, we claim that victory and accept the gift of forgiveness. Lord, there was another victory at the cross. You said that by Your stripes we are healed. We walk in that promise as well, knowing and understanding that healing is not always cure, but that it is the deepest healing of our hearts unto salvation. We thank You that every detail of our lives matter to You. You have a plan and purpose for _____'s life. We pray that Your destiny for him/her will be fulfilled. We ask that You would open the windows of heaven and pour out Your grace and mercy over his/her family as they walk through this health crisis/medical challenge. Comfort their hearts and fill them with peace.

In Jesus' name, Amen.

MINISTRY SERVICES/BLESSINGS/PRAYERS

Hospitals respect the ecumenical nature of their patient population and are generally most accommodating when this need is communicated to them. Do not hesitate in inviting the staff's participation when they are available.

If there is another patient in the room, provision needs to be made so there is no detrimental effect on them when ministering to the needs of the patient you are concerned about.

Spiritual gifts may be needed more than flowers, candy, balloons or stuffed animals. Here you will find other approaches to spiritual ministry that may have more far reaching results.

Anointing and Laying On of Hands

Roy Lawrence in his book *The Practice of Christian Healing* teaches on page 52, "Jesus expected his followers to incorporate the laying on of hands into the heart of the healing ministry they derived from Him. He said, 'Those who believe … will place their hands on sick people, and they will get well' (Mark 16:17-18). In other words, the Christian church, as the body of Christ, is not only to speak the Word of Christ but also to give the touch of Christ.

"It is worth noting that the prerequisite for laying on hands is not ordination to the clerical ministry or the possession of some special gift. It is simply belief—belief in Jesus as Savior and Lord, belief in his healing ministry, belief in the validity of its continuation in his body, the church."

In James 5:14 we are admonished to call the elders, anoint with oil, and make confession. It is assumed that those involved in the anointing service will have been encouraged to spend time with God in advance, doing some heart-searching and preparation, making sure that all is well between them and God and all sins are confessed.

For anointing with oil, you can use some fresh olive oil or purchase some anointing oil from a Book and Bible House. First consecrate it to God's service. Place your forefinger over the anointing bottle of oil and anoint the sufferer on the forehead. You can make the sign of the cross as you say, "I anoint you in the name of the Father, and of the Son, and of the Holy Spirit, that you might know the healing power of His love." Continue with a prayer claiming one or more of God's healing promises appropriate for the patient's needs, thanking God for hearing your prayer.

Put some thought into this sacred time. Following your tradition, be sure and make the anointing service special. You could sing some songs, read some scripture, or share a testimony. Each person participating can pray, or you alone can bless the patient. Be creative.

When the sun was setting, all those who had any that were sick with various diseases brought them to Him;

and He laid His hands on every one of them and healed them.—Luke 4:40

Is anyone among you sick? Let him call for the elders of the church, and let them pray over him, anointing him with oil in the name of the Lord. And the prayer of faith will save the sick, and the Lord will raise him up. And if he has committed sins, he will be forgiven.
—James 5:14-15

And they cast out many demons, and anointed with oil many who were sick, and healed them.—Mark 6:13

and begged Him earnestly saying, "My little daughter lies at the point of death. Come and lay Your hands on her that she may be healed, and she will live."—Mark 5:23

they will take up serpents; and if they drink anything deadly, it will by no means hurt them; they will lay hands on the sick, and they will recover."—Mark 16:18

When the sun was setting, all those who had any that were sick with various diseases brought them to Him; and He laid His hands on every one of them and healed them.—Luke 4:40

And it happened that the father of Publius lay sick of a fever and dysentery. Paul went in to him and prayed, and he laid his hands on him and healed him.—Acts 28:8

Baptism

It is rarely possible to do a baptism by immersion in the hospital unless the patient is mobile enough. If death is forthcoming and the dying person desires baptism, you may administer it by pouring water on their forehead or by doing a foot-washing ceremony, using the person's name, say, "I now baptize you in the name of the Father, the Son, and the Holy Spirit. Amen."

Communion/Sacred Symbols of Sacraments/Ordinances

Sacraments/Ordinances are acts which have meanings deeper than words because of what they symbolize and the longtime traditions attached to them. The mystical effect of communion, also referred to as the Eucharist, identifies with Christ and the Church. For the very spiritual/religious patient, the sacraments or spiritual symbols can symbolize their eternal future/destiny and is of significant importance that they be administered, particularly to the Catholic patient.

The grape juice/wine symbolizes Christ's sacrifice and cleansing blood, which offers forgiveness of sins and new beginnings. The bread/wafer, which symbolizes Christ's body, offers healing according to the text in Isaiah 53:4-5 which proclaims that the Lord took up our infirmities, carried our sorrows and by his stripes we are healed.

Communion may require permission from the doctor or nurse to be sure the patient can ingest the elements. Communicating with staff regarding the time you will be administrating sacraments, will provide needed privacy, which generally is respected, or an inclusion of staff members as appropriate. For the sacraments to be of greatest value to the patient, the person administering the service must understand what they mean to the patient at this time, in this specific experience. If the patient is unable to have the communion bread, you might ask the hospital chaplain if meltable wafers are available to place in the juice/wine.

This service is primarily to remove any obstacle between God and the patient, as they will spend time in repentance and confession prior to communion or sharing sacraments. It is important to assist the patient in dealing with forgiveness issues if necessary.

When the hour had come, He sat down, and the twelve apostles with Him. Then He said to them, "With fervent desire I have desired to eat this Passover with you before I suffer; for I say to you, I will no longer eat of it until it is fulfilled in the kingdom of God." Then He took the cup, and gave thanks, and said, "Take this and divide it among yourselves; for I say to you, I will not drink of the fruit of the vine until the kingdom of God comes." And He took bread, gave thanks and broke it, and gave it to them, saying, "This is My body which is given for you; do this in remembrance of Me." Likewise He also took the cup after supper, saying, "This cup is the new covenant in My blood, which is shed for you.—Luke 22:14-20

For I received from the Lord that which I also delivered to you: that the Lord Jesus on the same *night in which He was betrayed took bread; and when He had given thanks, He broke* it *and said, "Take, eat; this is My body which is broken for you; do this in remembrance of Me." In the same manner He also took the cup after supper, saying, "This cup is the new covenant in My blood. This do, as often as you drink* it, *in remembrance of Me." For as often as you eat this bread and drink this cup, you proclaim the Lord's death till He comes. Therefore whoever eats this bread or drinks* this *cup of the Lord in an unworthy manner will be guilty of the body and blood of the Lord. But let a man examine himself, and so let him eat of the bread and drink of the cup. For he who eats and drinks in an unworthy manner eats and drinks judgment to himself, not discerning the Lord's body. For this reason many* are *weak and sick among you, and many sleep. For if we would judge ourselves, we would not be judged. But when we are judged, we are chastened by the Lord, that we may not be condemned with the world.*—1 Corinthians 11:23-32

BLESSINGS

Childbirth/Child dedication or blessing

Then little children were brought to Him that He might put His *hands on them and pray, …*
—Matthew 19:13

This is a beautiful way of welcoming a new arrival, to celebrate an adoptive child into the family or honor an older child who has not yet received a blessing or been dedicated. If the parents are agreeable, hold the child in your arms as you pray over him (her). Incorporate one of the stories from the following texts in the blessing service. A favorite poem or quote from the family passed down as part of a legacy would be nice to include in the service as well. Parents seem to appreciate having the spiritual meaning of the child's name included. A good resource to use is *The Name Book* by Dorothy Astoria, ISBN 1-55661-982-0. Words of love and blessing should be summoned from God. He knows what His destiny is for this child and will gladly anoint your lips.

After reading the definition, prayer could be offered. Ask God's protection over the child. Ask that he/she will live to fulfill the meaning of her/his name, God's destiny. Verbalize the fact that this child is a gift from God entrusted to the parents to nurture and raise up for the Kingdom of God. Pray God's wisdom and unity over parents as they work together to raise this child.

Baby Dedication Certificates are sometimes available at the Chaplain/Spiritual Care department or you can create one on your computer.

You might have the guests write special messages or prayers on cards provided to leave with the parents. Follow up with a dedication certificate—purchased or created.

Prayer: Dear Lord, what a wonderful day this is. We are so thankful that You have blessed us with this treasure from heaven and we are all gathered here today to welcome him (her) with open arms and show our desire to support and encourage his (her) parents.

Today, we offer up this child in dedication. We give this baby (child) back to You and recognize _____ as a child of God. Please fill him (her) with the Holy Spirit to work in his (her) heart and direct his (her) thoughts. By Your grace and help we will love, protect, care for, teach and guide _____. May our example and influence guide _____ into living a righteous and honorable life drawing others to You.

We thank You in the precious name of Jesus, Amen.

At that time the disciples came to Jesus, saying, "Who then is greatest in the kingdom of heaven?" Then Jesus called a little child to Him, set him in the midst of them, and said, "Assuredly, I say to you, unless you are converted and become as little children, you will by no means enter the kingdom of heaven. Therefore whoever humbles himself as this little child is the greatest in the kingdom of heaven. Whoever receives one little child like this in My name receives Me.—Matthew 18:1-6

Then they brought little children to Him, that He might touch them; but the disciples rebuked those who brought them. *But when Jesus saw* it, *He was greatly displeased and said to them, "Let the little children come to Me, and do not forbid them; for of such is the kingdom of God. Assuredly, I say to you, whoever does not receive the kingdom of God as a little child will by no means enter it." And He took them up in His arms, laid* His *hands on them, and blessed them.*—Mark 10:13-16

And Mary said: "My soul magnifies the Lord, and my spirit has rejoiced in God my Savior. For He has regarded the lowly state of His maidservant; for behold, henceforth all generations will call me blessed. For He who is mighty has done great things for me, and holy is *His name."*—Luke 1:46-49

Healing Baskets and Supportive Actions

Family members who spend a considerable time in the hospital room with a failing or recovering patient often neglect their own needs. A basket of healthy snacks, encouraging notes, suitable reading material, games, books and toiletries is another way of saying, "We care." Include items that the patient might need as well.

Family members are pulled in many directions, just to keep up with life, as they stand by the patient. Church members can convey messages, send food, help care for other children, clean the house, and prepare it for the patient's return. All of this should be done with permission, so as to not embarrass or offend the family.

Music/Singing—Praise and Hymns-Rituals

Music is wonderfully soothing, encouraging, and healing. Whether the music is instrumental or vocal, whether spiritually produced in familiar hymns or contemporary praise, it can be uplifting and change the attitude and perspective of the patients as they become absorbed in it. It can be as effective to the unconscious patient as well, and give them reason to hold on to life or peacefully surrender to God's plan. Use music respectfully if the patient has a roommate.

The familiarity of sacred rituals can bring much peace to the patient and family. Sharing a meaningful and known prayer together, or other traditions of their faith, has the ability to decrease the patient's blood pressure and reduce an elevated heart rate. Dr. Herbert Benson ascertains that the relaxation response provides a direct linkage to faith in something beyond.

Prayer shows loving concern and is a means of bringing comfort, spiritual assurance, confidence in decision-making, and peace in the midst of the patient's health crisis. Prayer creates an atmosphere in which the presence of God is felt and where the Holy Spirit is invited to comfort, minister and guide. If applied sensitively and timely, it can also enhance the relationship between the patient and the intercessor. Be sure to ask the patient what they would like you to include in the prayer. Pray Scripture, there is power in the Word!

When praying do not seem like a "faith healer." Ultimately we must accept that God has a plan and purpose for each life. While death is an interruption of God's perfect plan, that we were to live forever, it is a reality of the consequences of sin and our life on this earth. In Isaiah 57:1-2 NIV we are instructed that *The righteous perish, and no one takes it to heart; the devout are taken away, and no one understands that the righteous are taken away to be spared from evil. Those who walk uprightly enter into peace; they find rest as they lie in death.* We do not know when it is the end of one's time on this earth. We can pray our heart, claim God's promises, and ask for God's will that His destiny for the patient be fulfilled.

In some cases it is okay if the patient chooses death. Be sensitive to the situation and to God's voice.

THE LORD'S PRAYER

… Our Father which art in heaven, Hallowed be thy name. Thy kingdom come, Thy will be done in earth, as it is in heaven. Give us this day our daily bread. And forgive us our debts as we forgive our debtors. And lead us not into temptation, but deliver us from evil: For thine is the kingdom, and the power, and the glory, for ever. Amen.

—Matthew 6:9-13 KJV

PATIENT'S PRAYER

God, thank You for seeing my pain and suffering and for providing people who care to minister to my needs. Help me to be faithful to You in this trial and thoughtful of others. May I trust in your promises and exemplify Christ in my suffering that I might receive the crown of life here and in eternity. In Jesus' name, Amen

PRAYER FOR PERSONAL HEALING

(Taken from *God's Word for your Healing,* p131)

Father, in the name of Jesus, I confess Your Word concerning healing. As I do this, I believe and say Your Word will not re-turn to You void, but will accomplish what it says it will. Therefore, I believe in the name of Jesus that I am healed, according to 1 Peter 2;24, *who Himself self bore our sins in His own body on the tree, that we, having died to sins, might live for righteousness—by whose stripes* [we] *were healed.* It is written in Your Word in Matthew 8;17, that Jesus took our infirmities and bore our sicknesses. Therefore, with great boldness and confidence I say on the authority of that written Word that I am redeemed from the curse of sickness, and I refuse to tolerate its symptoms.

I hold fast to my confession of faith; in Your Word I stand immovable and fixed in full assurance that I have health and healing now in the name of Jesus, Amen.

Prayer for Healing for Someone in Need

(Taken from *God's Word for your Healing,* p132-133)

Father, in Jesus' name, I pray and ask for a manifestation of Your healing power to flow into _____'s body right now. Father, Your Word tells us in James 5:16 to pray one for another that we might be healed. I believe, based

upon Your Word, that it is Your will that
_____ be made whole physically, men-
tally, and in every area of his/her life.

Father, as Your Word reads in Ephesians 1:18, I
ask that _____'s eyes be open to the
full understanding and knowledge that healing is
his/hers today. I pray that _____ will
have a complete revelation of Your healing
power and the redemptive work of Jesus upon
the cross for our healing.

I thank You now Father for healing
_____, in Jesus' name, Amen.

HEART DISEASE, PRAYER AND COUNSEL FOR

1. Break any family (generational) curses and
   command healing of other body parts af-
   fected.

2. Pray for a new heart.

   *I will give you a new heart and put a new spirit
   within you; I will take the heart of stone out of your
   flesh and give you a heart of flesh. I will put My
   Spirit within you and cause you to walk in My statutes, and you will keep My judgments and do
   them.*—Ezekiel 36:26-27

3. Love.

   *"Teacher, which is the great commandment in the
   law?" Jesus said to him, "You shall love the LORD*

your God with all your heart, with all your soul, and with all your mind.' This is the first and great commandment. And the second is like it: 'You shall love your neighbor as yourself.'

—Matthew 22:36-39

4. Look to the future.

Brethren, I do not count myself to have apprehended; but one thing I do, forgetting those things which are behind and reaching forward to those things which are ahead.—Philippians 3:13

BEFORE SURGERY (OR ANY PROCEDURE)

See also scripture verses you can include.

Heavenly Father, we come to you today in behalf of _____ who is facing surgery (a procedure). We ask that you will hand pick the medical staff who will be ministering to his/her needs. We pray that You will work through them with skill and expertise beyond themselves, that they too will know they have been touched by the hand of God. We ask that You will fill the room with ministering angels surrounding _____. If there is any hallucinating, may he/she hallucinate about the Lord Jesus Christ. We come against the spirit of fear and cover _____ with the armor of God that the devil may have no in-roads. We ask You to carry his/her pain and suffering/sorrow as You have promised and expedite the healing process. May _____ find comfort, courage, and peace in Your presence as he/she trusts in You.

In Jesus' name, Amen

PRAYER OF COMMITMENT

If the person is accepting Jesus as their Lord and Savior, have them repeat this prayer after you.

Dear Heavenly Father,

I believe Jesus Christ is Your only begotten Son. I believe He became a man and died on the cross, to pay the penalty for my sins that were separating me from You. I believe he was buried and rose from the dead physically, to give me new life.

Lord Jesus, I ask You to forgive my sins. I receive You as my Lord and Savior. I ask You to come into my heart. I believe You have forgiven my sins and have come into my heart. I thank You for Your promise of eternal life given in Your Word. John 3:36 says, *He who believes in the Son has everlasting life; and he who does not believe the Son shall not see life, but the wrath of God abides on him.* And in 2 Corinthians 5:17, *Therefore, if anyone is in Christ, he is a new creation; old things have passed away; behold, all things have become new.*

Thank You for Your sacrifice and victory. Thank You for Your love. Thank You that this is a time of new beginnings. I choose You and new life.

In Jesus' name, Amen

PRAYER CLOTH

Now God worked unusual miracles by the hands of Paul, so that even handkerchiefs or aprons were brought from his body to the sick, and the diseases left them and the evil spirits went out of them.—Acts 19:11-12

The *Bible* speaks only once about prayer cloth, but if it is mentioned even once, it is there for our benefit and blessing.

We have given a handkerchief or small 2x2 inch square cloth that we have laid hands on, anointed and prayed over asking God for a miracle of healing and life. They can be placed under the pillow or wherever they are needed. They can be mailed to loved ones or friends.

We rejoice that we have received testimonies of miracles.

PRAYER WALKING

Prayer walking is walking your community or any area of your community. For example you can prayer walk your church, the hospital, schools, businesses, etc. to bless and protect them. It is letting the Holy Spirit guide you for the prayer needs of that particular place and chatting with God spontaneously as those needs are revealed to your heart. You are talking, listening and interceding for specific needs for Kingdom purposes.

He has shown you, O man, what is good; And what does the LORD require of you But to do justly, To love mercy, And to walk humbly with your God?
—Micah 6:8

After the death of Moses the servant of the LORD, it came to pass that the LORD spoke to Joshua the son of Nun, Moses' assistant, saying: "Moses My servant is dead. Now therefore, arise, go over this Jordan, you and all this people, to the land which I am giving to them— the children of Israel. Every place that the sole of your foot will tread upon I have given you, as I said to Moses. Then you shall rise from the ambush and seize the city, for the LORD your God will deliver it into your hand. So Moses swore on that day, saying, 'Surely the land where your foot has trodden shall be your inheritance and your children's forever, because you have wholly followed the LORD my God.—Joshua 1:1-3,8:7,14:9

Death, Supportive Readings at Time of

The LORD is my shepherd; I shall not want. He makes me to lie down in green pastures; He leads me beside the still waters. He restores my soul; He leads me in the paths of righteousness For His name's sake. Yea, though I walk through the valley of the shadow of death, I will fear no evil; For You are with me; Your rod and Your staff, they comfort me. You prepare a table before me in the presence of my enemies; You anoint my head with oil; My cup runs over. Surely goodness and mercy shall follow me All the days of my life; And I will dwell in the house of the LORD Forever.—Psalm 23

Thou dost guide me with thy counsel, and afterward thou wilt receive me to glory. Whom have I in heaven but thee? And there is nothing upon earth that I desire besides thee. My flesh and my heart may fail, but God is the strength of my heart and my portion for ever.
—Psalm 73:24-26 RSV

I love the LORD, because He has heard My voice and my supplications. Because He has inclined His ear to me, Therefore I will call upon Him as long as I live. The pains of death surrounded me, And the pangs of Sheol laid hold of me; I found trouble and sorrow. Then I called upon the name of the LORD: "O LORD, I implore You, deliver my soul!" Gracious is the LORD, and righteous; Yes, our God is merciful. The LORD preserves the simple; I was brought low, and He saved me. Return to your rest, O my soul, For the LORD has dealt bounti-

209

fully with you. For You have delivered my soul from death, My eyes from tears, And my feet from falling. I will walk before the LORD *In the land of the living. O* LORD, *truly I am Your servant; I am Your servant, the son of Your maidservant; You have loosed my bonds.*
—Psalm 116:1-9,16

"I will ransom them from the power of the grave; I will redeem them from death. O Death, I will be your plagues! O Grave, I will be your destruction! Pity is hidden from My eyes."—Hosea 13:14

And as Moses lifted up the serpent in the wilderness, even so must the Son of Man be lifted up, that whoever believes in Him should not perish but have eternal life. For God so loved the world that He gave His only begotten Son, that whoever believes in Him should not perish but have everlasting life.—John 3:14-16

Peace I leave with you, My peace I give to you; not as the world gives do I give to you. Let not your heart be troubled, neither let it be afraid.—John 14:27

"Let not your heart be troubled; you believe in God, believe also in Me. In My Father's house are many mansions; if it were *not so, I would have told you. I go to prepare a place for you. And if I go and prepare a place for you, I will come again and receive you to Myself; that where I am,* there *you may be also.*—John 14:1-3

Who shall separate us from the love of Christ? Shall tribulation, or distress, or persecution, or famine, or nakedness, or peril, or sword? As it is written: "For Your sake we are killed all day long; we are accounted as sheep for the slaughter." Yet in all these things we are more than conquerors through Him who loved us. For I am persuaded that neither death nor life, nor angels nor principalities nor powers, nor things present nor things to come, nor height nor depth, nor any other created thing, shall be able to separate us from the love of God which is in Christ Jesus our Lord.—Romans 8:35-39

But we have this treasure in earthen vessels, that the excellence of the power may be of God and not of us. We are hard-pressed on every side, yet not crushed; we are perplexed, but not in despair; persecuted, but not forsaken; struck down, but not destroyed—always carrying about in the body the dying of the Lord Jesus, that the life of Jesus also may be manifested in our body. For we who live are always delivered to death for Jesus' sake, that the life of Jesus also may be manifested in our mortal flesh. So then death is working in us, but life in you. And since we have the same spirit of faith, according to what is written, "I believed and therefore I spoke," we also believe and therefore speak, knowing that He who raised up the Lord Jesus will also raise us up with Jesus, and will present us with you. For all things are for your sakes, that grace, having spread through the many, may cause thanksgiving to abound to the glory of God. Therefore we do not lose heart. Even though our outward man is perishing, yet the inward man is being renewed day by day. For our light affliction, which is but for a moment, is working for us a far more exceeding and eternal weight of glory, while we do not look at the things which are seen, but at the things which are not seen. For the things *which are seen* are *temporary, but the things which are not seen* are *eternal.*—2 Corinthians 4:7-18

For if we believe that Jesus died and rose again, even so God will bring with Him those who sleep in Jesus. For this we say to you by the word of the Lord, that we who are alive and *remain until the coming of the Lord will by no means precede those who are asleep. For the Lord Himself will descend from heaven with a shout, with the voice of an archangel, and with the trumpet of God. And the dead in Christ will rise first. Then we who are alive* and *remain shall be caught up together with them in the clouds to meet the Lord in the air. And thus we shall always be with the Lord. Therefore comfort one another with these words."*—1 Thessalonians 4:14-18

Now I saw a new heaven and a new earth, for the first heaven and the first earth had passed away. Also there was no more sea. Then I, John, saw the holy city, New Jerusalem, coming down out of heaven from God, prepared as a bride adorned for her husband. And I heard a loud voice from heaven saying, "Behold, the tabernacle of God is with men, and He will dwell with them, and they shall be His people. God Himself will be with them and be their God. And God will wipe away every tear from their eyes; there shall be no more death, nor sorrow, nor crying. There shall be no more pain, for the former things have passed away." Then He who sat on the throne said, "Behold, I make all things new." And He said to me, "Write, for these words are true and faithful."—Revelations 21:1-5

INFANT/CHILD'S DEATH

Then she went and sat down across from him *at a distance of about a bowshot; for she said to herself, "Let me not see the death of the boy." So she sat opposite* him, *and lifted her voice and wept. And God heard the voice of the lad. Then the angel of God called to Hagar out of heaven, and said to her, "What ails you, Hagar? Fear not, for God has heard the voice of the lad where he* is. *"Arise, lift up the lad and hold him with your hand, for I will make him a great nation." Then God opened her eyes, and she saw a well of water. And she went and filled the skin with water, and gave the lad a drink. So God was with the lad; and he grew and dwelt in the wilderness, and became an archer.*—Genesis 21:16-20

And he went up and lay on the child, and put his mouth on his mouth, his eyes on his eyes, and his hands on his hands; and he stretched himself out on the child, and the flesh of the child became warm.—2 Kings 4:34

For You formed my inward parts; You covered me in my mother's womb. I will praise You, for I am fearfully and *wonderfully made; Marvelous are Your works, And* that *my soul knows very well.*—Psalm 139:13-14

Thus says the LORD: *"A voice was heard in Ramah, Lamentation* and *bitter weeping, Rachel weeping for her children, Refusing to be comforted for her children, Because they* are *no more."*—Jeremiah 31:15

INFANT DEATH PRAYERS

Dear Lord, we do not know why this precious treasure is gone from us. We do not understand why so many of our hopes and dreams have now been dashed. Our hearts cry out to you in pain and question.

Today we recognize the fragility of the gift of life. Our expectations have turned to heartache and disappointment. As our hearts cry out, as our arms are empty, we pray for grace and mercy to help us walk in the power of faith through this trial and keep us close to you. We pray that You will wrap us in Your arms of love and hold us close to Your heart. We pray that Your tears will mingle with ours and Your comfort will be poured out abundantly. May Your presence and love engulf us.

In Jesus' blessed name, Amen.

Prayer: adapted from 2 Corinthians 1:3-4:

Blessed be our God who consoles us in our affliction, so that we, by grace may be able to console those who are in any affliction with the consolations with which we ourselves are consoled by God.

Prayer for Those Grieving

O Holy One, Our Father and Our God, teach us how to grieve. Give us the courage to acknowledge our pain, to hold it awhile and then to set it free. Give us the strength to choose to move beyond what has altered our life forever, to find a new normal; a new life where precious memories bring gladness. Help us to honor new beginnings by building upon our memories a life of joy and hope. We will be gentle with ourselves and with each other during this process and take time to grieve and heal. Thank you for carrying us through this journey. In Jesus' name, Amen.

—Karen Johnston

Prayer of Surrender

My Father and my God,

You are greater than all life's problems, greater than heartache and pain. When the world and its troubles are remembered no more, Your love will always remain. I know that by simply asking, You will walk beside me all the way. Please take my hand and help me trust in You and surrender to Your divine and perfect plan for my life.

In Jesus' name, Amen.

Be joyful in hope, patient in affliction, faithful in prayer.—Romans 12:12

God's love for us is not a love that always exempts us from trials, but rather, a love that sees us through trials.

—Unknown

It is the LORD who goes before you. He will be with you; he will not leave you or forsake you. Do not fear or be dismayed."—Deuteronomy 31:8

If we are not in the habit of praying, it is often the last place we go for help. But God wants us to have confidence in approaching Him; and as we present our requests, He promises that if we call on Him, He will listen.

—Derry

'Call to me and I will answer you and tell you great and unsearchable things you do not know.'
—Jeremiah 33:3

Meaningful Funerals/Memorial Services

- Meaningful services include all close family members in the planning process.

- It is important to remember that the services are for the survivors acknowledging the death of someone they love.

- The service is a way for them to focus on those things that were noteworthy about their loved one. It opens the opportunity for support from caring people.

- Each service can be unique and distinctive according to the needs of the family. Comfort and meaning from traditional ceremonies can still reflect the unique personality of the family and the person who died. Adding personal touches to even traditional services can make the service one that will be remembered and appreciated. (See the following examples.)

- Give the family the freedom to ask friends and other family members to be involved in the service. They can share responsibilities or participate in activities such as special readings, writing and reading the eulogy, special music, or inviting attendees to share memories.

- Encourage the family and close friends to view the body before entering the service. Many people find this helps them acknowledge the reality of the death. It also provides a way to say goodbye. There is nothing morbid or wrong about this practice.

- Another effective and consoling goodbye gift is to have a bouquet of roses or other preferred flowers at the graveside. Pass them out to family members to lie on top of the casket. You can invite them to place flowers there at the end of your service. You can also invite them to pray a favorite prayer or cherish a memory as they place their flowers.

- Encourage survivors to embrace their feelings and openly express them. There is no shame in crying.

- The service should also reflect the spirituality of the families and the deceased. If there is any question what direction to take, lean towards the spirituality of the deceased. (Unless they were not Christian and you have an audience of many Christians or seekers.) Help survivors to find comfort in their faith through the service.

- Frequently when a loved one dies, the survivors might find themselves questioning their faith, and the very meaning of life and death. This is natural. Encourage the search for meaning. Do not let others dismiss this journey with clichéd responses, such as, "It was God's will" or "Think of what you still have to be thankful for."

- Make use of memories during the service. Fun, personal memories can be included in the eulogy to make it more interesting, and draw more people in. Memories are part of the best legacies that exist after the death of someone loved. Stress the word "legacy" and what the deceased is leaving behind for the family to hang on to and live out in their lives. Ask those attending the funeral to share their most special memory of the person who died.

- Some people are reticent about sharing in a group setting. Encourage sharing at the reception following. Encourage visitors to share particular memories of the deceased that would become a treasure to the hearer.

- If you are not familiar with the deceased, after reading or hearing the eulogy and listening to the stories shared, a nice thing to say is, "I wish I had known _____. I think we would have been good friends."

- Consider closing by reading the poem "The Dash" by Linda Ellis: https://lindaellis.life/the-dash-poem and make an appeal.

- Give them a very small box (like a jewelry box—bracelet sized) wrapped in shiny gold paper. Tell them, "This is a 'Memory Box,' not to be opened but to remind you of cherished memories."

- Suggest they plant a tree or flowering shrub in their yard in memory of their loved one, or establish a Memory Garden area.

- For some, it is beneficial to have them write the deceased a letter. Encourage them to share their feelings, even to say, "I'm angry with you for leaving me." Have them write memories, words of thanks, dreams that will go unfulfilled, and their love. They can place this letter in the casket, put it away until the first year anniversary of death, or until they want to re-read it, if ever.

Caution: Do not assume that people will want to memorialize the date of death. Some families would rather not be reminded of this heartache every year. They will never forget their loved one. There will be memories forever tucked in their minds and hearts. They will see their loved one in the faces and mannerisms of other family members; but to have an appointed day for grieving is debilitating to them.

God is Love. We are called to love one another as He loves us.

May God abundantly bless you as you minister to those who need you, or if you are the patient—give you the courage and peace to journey through this challenge.

Titles by Dr. Derry James-Tannariello

For gift or bulk orders of these, or any of Derry's books, please visit our website:

FreedomInSurrender.net

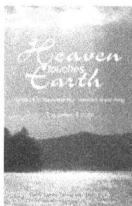

Heaven Touches Earth— Handbook for Supporting Sick, Terminally Ill and Dying, Expanded Edition *was written to provide you with the skills and tools necessary to bring solace and comfort to the sick and suffering at home, in the hospital or hospice ministry.*

This concise how-to handbook is also a succinct resource of clear insight into hospital practices and protocols useful in training volunteers, parish visitors, pastors and chaplains and a helpful refresher guide for those who have studied hospital ministry.

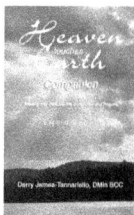

Heaven Touches Earth Companion—Healing and Deliverance Scriptures and Prayers, Expanded Edition *is a take-along resource containing only the Healing and Deliverance Scriptures and Prayers chapters of the* Heaven Touches Earth *book. It is designed for those ministering in a supportive role.*

Also available in eBook format at Amazon.com, or at

FreedomInSurrender.net

Living Volumes One and Two:

Praying in the "YES" of God

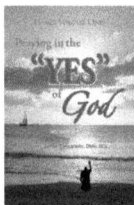

God knows your name! *Do you believe that? Do you believe there even is a God?*

Do you believe Jesus Christ knows who you are and is interested in your life? Do you believe He is Who He says He is, and can do what He says He can do?

When you pray, does it sometimes feel like your prayers are hitting the ceiling, or are falling on deaf ears? Are you angry with God because your prayers seem not to be answered? Have you given up asking God for things for yourself because you don't want to be disappointed again; or you're afraid if God is silent you will begin to question His existence, and then you'll have nothing to put your hope and trust in?

Praying in the "YES" of God *will help you find those answers and give you the tools to face the unknown with the peace and confidence that God loves you! Learn how to live with triumphant faith, peace of mind, and enthusiastic testimony.*

Growing in the "YES" of God

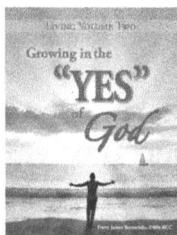

God Has a Plan for Your Life! *Do you wonder why it seems some people have answers to their prayers and unexplainable miracles in their life—and you don't? Is there really any such thing as security and joy? What does love mean? What if you could find the answers to these questions and more? You can.*

This in-depth Bible Study on principles of a more effective prayer life, further growth in Jesus and living out His character and plans for your life victoriously and blessed will reassure you of God's love. It is best understood and most effective if preceded by Living Volume One: Praying in the "YES" of God.

Also available in eBook format at Amazon.com, or at

FreedomInSurrender.net

Three Companion books:

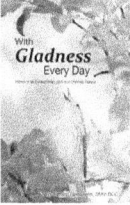

With Gladness Every Day

Become confident in your walk with God and ***increase your trust and hope in Him.*** *The stories in this book are answers to prayers and lessons from life experiences dependent on God's grace and mercy.*

In this time of uncertainty and turmoil in our nation, are you mindful of the magnificence of God's love and the countless ways He expresses it to you each day? If not, it's time to reconnect to God's presence and awaken your senses to His unconditional, all encompassing love for **you***.*

Be inspired by these stories, and let them arouse in you a desire to become acquainted with this King of kings, or renew your desire to commit all to Him and sing His praises!!!

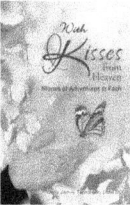

With Kisses from Heaven

Even in times of uncertainty, love produces a heart of gratitude. *With a thankful and adoring heart we notice the small as well as the larger things done for us—out of love and devotion to us.*

God is continually doing and giving for us; for our best interest, for our delight, for our care and pleasure—to offer encouragement, protection and provision, or make life easier.

But always, always, it is to let us know He is there, right by our side, attentive and aware of everything that concerns us, pouring out love in unexpected ways. I call these surprises "Kisses from Heaven."

I pray that by sharing some of my experiences of God's intervention and lessons learned that punctuate particular Scriptures, you will become more aware of how attentive God is to **you***. May your heart burst with appreciation and may your love for Him increase. May your faith grow and keep you steadfast when the trials of life attempt to overwhelm you.*

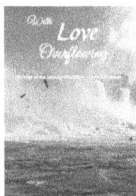

With Love Overflowing

God's abiding love is ever present. He offers a place of peace, hope for the future and freedom from fear. *Every day is a new day of life and opportunities; challenges and joys. In this world of insecurity, we are looking for dependable security and unconditional love. The nature of life is such that conflict—inner and outer—is inevitable. Can we find peace, security and love amidst conflict? The answer is Yes! We can find it all in the overflowing love of God in Christ Jesus.*

I pray these stories will open your eyes to the many ways God has proven Himself present in your life and confirm there is hope in Jesus during life's turmoil and storms. Our God of love is a personal, caring God Who loves extravagantly with overwhelming, incomprehensible love. He pours out His love on us and will use us to let others experience His love through us. He is there for you, even in silence. When you become aware of that, He will become irresistible to you too and you will desire to be more like Him.

Also available in eBook format at Amazon.com, or at

FreedomInSurrender.net

Upcoming Title
Fill My Life, Lord

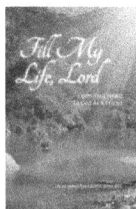

*What **fills** your mind, your heart, your home and your life depends upon what you allow to **fill** your hands.*

The stories in the Bible are not just stories to inspire and encourage you, but stories to build your relationship with God and change your life. What He has done in the past He will do for you in the present.

*If you don't have a personal relationship with God, I invite you to **fill** your hands with this book and open your mind and heart to this study. The Lord is waiting and willing to **fill** your life and prove He knows you and hears you. When you take one step towards the Savior, He runs the rest of the way to meet you. May your life be transformed.*

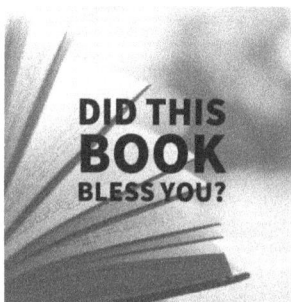

Why Not Bless Others!!!

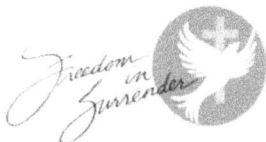

DID THIS BOOK BLESS YOU?

FreedomInSurrender.net

- ✓ Mention this book on your social media platforms.
- ✓ Are you a blogger? Consider writing a book review on your blog. Post it to your blog and other retail book outlets.
- ✓ Know someone else who would be blessed by this book? Pick up a copy for a friend or coworker.
- ✓ Recommend this book to your church library or small group study.
- ✓ Share this message on Facebook. "I was blessed by **Heaven Touches Earth** by Derry James-Tannariello and Freedom In Surrender Ministries."

Scan this QR code for
FreedomInSurrender.net

Or email Derry:
Derry@FreedomInSurrender.net

www.ingramcontent.com/pod-product-compliance
Lightning Source LLC
Chambersburg PA
CBHW051951090426
42741CB00008B/1347